Evidence-Based Review in Policy and Practice

Editor

ALAN PEARSON

NURSING CLINICS
OF NORTH AMERICA

www.nursing.theclinics.com

Consulting Editor
STEPHEN D. KRAU

December 2014 • Volume 49 • Number 4

ELSEVIER

1600 John F. Kennedy Boulevard • Suite 1800 • Philadelphia, Pennsylvania, 19103-2899

http://www.theclinics.com

NURSING CLINICS OF NORTH AMERICA Volume 49, Number 4
December 2014 ISSN 0029-6465, ISBN-13: 978-0-323-32662-9

Editor: Kerry Holland
Developmental Editor: Casey Jackson

Nursing Clinics of North America (ISSN 0029-6465) is published quarterly by Elsevier Inc., 360 Park Avenue South, New York, NY 10010-1710. Months of issue are March, June, September, and December. Periodicals postage paid at New York, NY and additional mailing offices. Subscription price per year is, $150.00 (US individuals), $400.00 (US institutions), $275.00 (international individuals), $488.00 (international institutions), $220.00 (Canadian individuals), $488.00 (Canadian institutions), $85.00 (US students), and $135.00 (international students). To receive student/resident rate, orders must be accompanied by name of affiliated institution, date of term, and the signature of program/residency coordinator on institution letterhead. Orders will be billed at individual rate until proof of status is received. Foreign air speed delivery is included in all *Clinics* subscription prices. All prices are subject to change without notice. **POSTMASTER:** Send address changes to *Nursing Clinics*, Elsevier Health Sciences Division, Subscription Customer Service, 3251 Riverport Lane, Maryland Heights, MO 63043. **Customer Service: Telephone: 1-800-654-2452** (U.S. and Canada); **1-314-447-8871 (outside U.S. and Canada). Fax: 1-314-447-8029. E-mail: journalscustomerservice-usa@elsevier.com** (for print support) and **journalsonlinesupport-usa@elsevier.com** (for online support).

Nursing Clinics of North America is covered in *EMBASE/Excerpta Medica, MEDLINE/PubMed (Index Medicus), Social Sciences Citation Index, Current Contents, ASCA, Cumulative Index to Nursing, RNdex Top 100,* and Allied Health Literature and International Nursing Index (INI).

Printed in the United States of America.

Contributors

CONSULTING EDITOR

STEPHEN D. KRAU, PhD, RN, CNE
Associate Professor, Vanderbilt University Medical Center, School of Nursing, Nashville, Tennessee

EDITOR

ALAN PEARSON, AM, RN, ONC, DipNEd, DANS, MSc, PhD, FCNA, FAAG, FAAN, FRCN
Emeritus Professor of Evidence-Based Healthcare, The Joanna Briggs Institute, School of Translational Health Science, Faculty of Health Sciences, The University of Adelaide, Adelaide, South Australia, Australia

AUTHORS

JEF ADRIAENSSENS, RN, MSc
Deputy Director, Belgian Interuniversity Collaboration for Evidence-Based Practice (BICEP), Joanna Briggs Collaboration; Centre for Evidence-Based Medicine (CEBAM), Belgian Branch of the Dutch Cochrane Centre, Leuven, Belgium; PhD-Student, Health Psychology Unit, Institute of Psychology, Leiden University, Leiden, The Netherlands; Coordinator, Platform Science and Practice, Brussels, Belgium; Member of Board of Directors, EBMPracticenet, Brussels, Belgium

EDOARDO AROMATARIS, BSc, PhD
Associate Professor, Faculty of Health Sciences, The Joanna Briggs Institute, Director Synthesis Science, School of Translational Health Science, The University of Adelaide, Adelaide, South Australia, Australia

FIONA BATH-HEXTALL, PhD
Professor of Evidence Based Health Care, School of Health Sciences, Queen's Medical Centre, University of Nottingham, Nottingham, United Kingdom

CELIA MARIA SIVALLI CAMPOS, RN, MSc (Nursing), PhD
Associate Professor, Department of Collective Health Nursing, School of Nursing, University of São Paulo, São Paulo, Brazil

MABEL FERNANDES FIGUEIRO, Bachelor (Library Sciences)
General Coordination Center of Health Technology Assessment, Hospital do Coração/HCor, São Paulo, Brazil

ERIK FRANCK, RN, PhD
Department of Health Care, Lecturer, Karel de Grote University College; Faculty of Medicine and Health Sciences, Professor, Centre for Research and Innovation in Care (CRIC), University of Antwerp, Antwerp, Belgium

BART GEURDEN, RN, PhD
Department of Health Care, Lecturer, Karel de Grote University College; Faculty of Medicine and Health Sciences, Academic Assistant and PhD-Student, Centre for Research and Innovation in Care (CRIC), University of Antwerp, Antwerp, Belgium; Director, Belgian Interuniversity Collaboration for Evidence-Based Practice (BICEP), Joanna Briggs Collaboration Affiliated Centre; Member of Staff, Centre for Evidence-Based Medicine(CEBAM), Belgian Branch of the Dutch Cochrane Centre, Leuven, Belgium

CHERYL HOLLY, EdD, RN, ANEF
Co-Director, Northeast Institute for Evidence Translation and Synthesis; Associate Dean and Professor, Rutgers School of Nursing, Newark, New Jersey

LISA HOPP, PhD, RN, FAAN
Interim Dean, College of Nursing, Director, Indiana Center for Evidence Based Nursing Practice, Purdue University Calumet, Hammond, Indiana

CRAIG LOCKWOOD, RN, BN, GDipClinN, MNSc, PhD
Associate Professor, Faculty of Health Sciences; Director, Implementation Science, The Joanna Briggs Institute; Postgraduate Coordinator, School of Translational Health Science, The University of Adelaide, Adelaide, South Australia, Australia

ZACHARY MUNN, BMedRad(NucMed), GDHSc, PhD
Senior Research Fellow, Faculty of Health Sciences, Implementation Science, The Joanna Briggs Institute, School of Translational Health Science, The University of Adelaide, Adelaide, South Australia, Australia

ALAN PEARSON, AM, RN, ONC, DipNEd, DANS, MSc, PhD, FCNA, FAAG, FAAN, FRCN
Emeritus Professor of Evidence-Based Healthcare, The Joanna Briggs Institute, School of Translational Health Science, Faculty of Health Sciences, The University of Adelaide, Adelaide, South Australia, Australia

DRU RIDDLE, DNP, CRNA
Assistant Professor of Professional Practice and Associate Director, TCU Center of Evidence Based Practice and Research: A Collaborating Center of the Joanna Briggs Institute, School of Nurse Anesthesia, Texas Christian University — Harris College of Nursing and Health Sciences, Fort Worth, Texas

SUZANNE ROBERTSON-MALT, PhD
Director, Implementation Science, Joanna Briggs Institute, School of Translational Health Science, University of Adelaide, Adelaide, South Australia, Australia

SUSAN W. SALMOND, EdD, RN, ANEF, FAAN
Co-Director, Northeast Institute for Evidence Translation and Synthesis; Executive Vice Dean and Professor, Rutgers School of Nursing, Newark, New Jersey

JANE SMITH, DNP, RN, CNS
Morristown Memorial Hospital, Ortho/Trauma, Morristown, New Jersey

CASSIA BALDINI SOARES, RN, MPH, PhD
Associate Professor, Department of Collective Health Nursing, School of Nursing, University of São Paulo, São Paulo, Brazil

DAPHNE STANNARD, PhD, RN, CNS
Director and Chief Nurse Researcher, Institute for Nursing Excellence, Director, UCSF Centre for Evidence-Based Patient and Family Care: An Affiliate Centre if the Joanna Briggs Institute, Co-Chair, Surgical Services Node, Joanna Briggs Institute, University of California San Francisco Medical Center, San Francisco, California

SUSAN MACE WEEKS, DNP, RN, CNS, LMFT, FAAN, FNAP
Professor, Associate Dean of Nursing and Health Innovation, Texas Christian University – Harris College of Nursing and Health Sciences; Director, TCU Center for Evidence Based Practice and Research: A Collaborating Center of the Joanna Briggs Institute, Fort Worth, Texas

TATIANA YONEKURA, RN, MSc (Nursing)
PhD student, The Nursing Graduate Program (PPGE), School of Nursing, University of São Paulo, São Paulo, Brazil

Contents

Foreword: The Utilization of Evidenced-based Practice in Nursing: Some Important Considerations   xi

Stephen D. Krau

Preface: Evidence-based Nursing: Synthesizing the Best Available Evidence to Translate into Action in Policy and Practice   xiii

Alan Pearson

Evidence Synthesis and Its Role in Evidence-Based Health Care   453

Alan Pearson

> The central role of evidence synthesis (or the systematic review of evidence) in evidence-based health care is often poorly understood. There are numerous examples in the literature of poorly conceived and/or executed systematic reviews and of a lack of awareness of the international standards developed by the international leaders in systematic reviews. The Cochrane Collaboration has played a critical global role in developing and refining systematic review methods in relation to evidence of effects and of diagnostic accuracy.

The Systematic Review of Health Care Evidence: Methods, Issues, and Trends   461

Fiona Bath-Hextall

> The systematic review is a key component to the evidence based health care cycle. There are two main types of systematic reviews: qualitative and quantitative. Systematic reviews bring together large amounts of information that can help support individual patient decision, inform guidelines, policy and primary research. The basic steps for each type of systematic review are the same; however, differences occur in the tools used to appraise the included studies and the method of synthesis. Over the years, many different systems have been used to grade the quality (level) of evidence and the strength of recommendations, which has meant that the same evidence and recommendation could be graded differently according to the system used at the time.

Developing a Robust Evidence Base for Nursing   475

Lisa Hopp

> Systematic reviews provide robust evidence for nursing practice because of the exhaustiveness of search, the critical appraisal methods to determine the risks of bias, and synthesis methods that pool evidence to increase the power of statistical estimates or credibility of aggregated metasynthesis of qualitative findings. More consistency in publication standards will enhance the rigor of available evidence and allow nursing to live up to the promise of best available evidence.

Evidence in Perioperative Care   485

Dru Riddle and Daphne Stannard

> Perioperative care is comprised of preoperative, intraoperative, and post-operative care. Given the vulnerable status of the perioperative patient, coupled with the complex nature of these areas, evidence-based practice and clinical decision-making must be rooted in high-quality evidence for safe and effective patient and family care. Evidence-based practice is comprised of patient and family preferences, clinical expertise, and best available evidence. This article showcases systematic reviews that have focused on clinical issues within the preoperative, intraoperative, and postoperative care areas. A case study presents the importance of applying best available evidence to solve a thorny clinical problem and improve patient outcomes.

Evidence-Based Health Care in Pediatrics   493

Suzanne Robertson-Malt

> This article examines current trends in the type and quality of systematic reviews underpinning the evidence base for pediatric health care. A case study is used to highlight the quality standards for the conduct and publication of systematic reviews and the processes being used to transition the evidence produced from systematic reviews into the everyday systems and processes of care.

Finding and Using Best Evidence for Rehabilitation   507

Susan W. Salmond, Cheryl Holly, and Jane Smith

> With the demands for improved experiences of care, improved outcomes, and greater efficiency/lower costs, the need for an evidence-based approach to care in rehabilitation settings has never been more urgent. This article guides practitioners in how to find the best available evidence for rehabilitation settings. It then discusses the use of evidence from systematic reviews through a high-impact case study: delirium in patients with postoperative hip fracture.

Evidence in Mental Health   525

Susan Mace Weeks

> Health practitioners wishing to positively improve health outcomes for their clients have access to a unique set of collated tools to guide their practice. Systematic reviews provide guidance in the form of synthesized evidence that can form the basis of decision making as they provide care for their clients. This article describes systematic reviews as a basis for informed decision making by mental health practitioners. The process of systematic review is discussed, examples of existing systematic review topics relevant to mental health are presented, a sample systematic review is described, and gaps and emerging topics for mental health systematic reviews are addressed.

Evidence in Public Health: Steps to Make It Real   **533**

Cassia Baldini Soares, Tatiana Yonekura, Celia Maria Sivalli Campos, and
Mabel Fernandes Figueiro

> This study addresses the methodological trends in the development of
> systematic reviews in public health, and examines the reviews of the
> Cochrane Public Health Group in order to exemplify syntheses of evidence
> in public health and its implementation and impact on practice and
> research.

Impact of Evidence and Health Policy on Nursing Practice   **545**

Bart Geurden, Jef Adriaenssens, and Erik Franck

> The story of evidence-based practice in nursing is long, with many
> successes, contributors, leaders, scientists, and enthusiasts. Nurse edu-
> cators have great advantages offered from a wide variety of educational
> resources for evidence-based practice. These resources offer students
> the opportunity to connect their emerging competencies with clinical
> needs for best practices in clinical and microsystem changes.

Translating Evidence into Policy and Practice   **555**

Craig Lockwood, Edoardo Aromataris, and Zachary Munn

> This paper uses a published case study to illustrate the practical applica-
> tion of a translational model for the implementation of evidence into prac-
> tice. The paper examines a translational approach to moving knowledge
> from robust methods for systematic review into guidance for clinical prac-
> tice, and then in to action followed by evaluation of its impact on practice
> and health care outcomes. The conceptual model for evidence-based
> health care reported in this paper provides the theoretic framework for
> practice change.

Index   **567**

Evidence-Based Review in Policy and Practice

NURSING CLINICS OF NORTH AMERICA

FORTHCOMING ISSUES

March 2015
**Transformational Toolkit for
Front Line Nurses**
Francisca Chita Farrar, *Editor*

June 2015
Technology in Nursing
Maria Overstreet, *Editor*

September 2015
**The Role of the Nurse in Mass Casualty
Incidents**
Robert W. Koch, *Editor*

RECENT ISSUES

September 2014
Integrating Evidence into Practice for Impact
Debra D. Mark, Marita G. Titler, and
Rene'e W. Latimer, *Editors*

June 2014
**Facilitating Aging in Place: Safe, Sound,
and Secure**
Barbara J. Holtzclaw and
Lazelle E. Benefield, *Editors*

March 2014
**Nursing-Sensitive Innovations in
Patient Care**
Cecilia Anne Kennedy Page, *Editor*

Foreword

The Utilization of Evidenced-based Practice in Nursing: Some Important Considerations

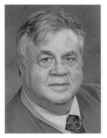

Stephen D. Krau, PhD, RN, CNE
Consulting Editor

What can be asserted without evidence can also be dismissed without evidence.
— *Christopher Hitchens*

The development of evidence-based practice (EBP) as a systematic approach to practice was initiated by Dr Archie Cochrane, a British epidemiologist, who was concerned about the efficacy of health care. He encouraged the public to pay for care that had been empirically demonstrated as being effective. Cochrane advocated for the use of rigorous research so that health care practitioners, policymakers, and health care institutions could make sound decisions.[1] As a result of Dr Cochrane's initiative and challenge for continued updated clinical trials, the Cochrane Center was opened in Oxford, England in 1992, and the Cochrane Collaboration was founded in 1993. The purpose of the Cochrane Collaboration, as a global independent network of health practitioners, researchers, patient advocates, and others, is to offer vast amounts of evidence generated through research that is practical for contributing to decisions about health.[2] The United Kingdom and Australia have been leaders in the implementation of EBP. This is largely due to the uniformity of health care systems, regulatory agencies, schools of medicine, schools of nursing, and government involved in health care in these countries. EBP has rapidly become a focus for health care systems in the United States.

Owing much to the initiatives of Dr Cochrane, the nursing profession has developed a system of international reviews that guide nursing practice across many topics. Information about the databases can be found through *Worldviews on Evidence-based Nursing* by Sigma Theta Tau International.[3] The purpose of the reviews is to contribute to the development of clinical practice guidelines that are based on the best evidence of specific topics.

Nurs Clin N Am 49 (2014) xi–xii
http://dx.doi.org/10.1016/j.cnur.2014.09.002
0029-6465/14/$ – see front matter © 2014 Elsevier Inc. All rights reserved.
nursing.theclinics.com

When utilizing evidence, it remains imperative that nurses continue to use a nursing perspective that respects the dignity, worth, and desires of each patient. Clearly, the goal of Evidenced-based Nursing is to make practice less subjective and increase the accountability that provides a stronger foundation on which to make clinical decisions. It remains problematic that there can be gaps in information and that certain patients or problems may present with issues not discerned in aggregate research findings. There are standard nursing and medical practices in which there is ongoing research and currently insufficient research. In addition, it has been proposed that the movement of EBP in nursing has become so pervasive that it is possible for nurses to fail to consider it with the same critical perspective as research in general.[4]

The utilization of EBP is an ongoing initiative that involves a broader approach to promoting acceptance of EBP, including strategies to correct misperceptions about EBP, and the development of skills. These skills can be achieved through educational endeavors such as workshops, conferences, publications, and handouts. The most effective learning method incorporates the teaching of didactic material in conjunction with interactive behavioral skills. Ongoing development of EBP is contingent on the health care professionals to explore practice questions.

It should not be forgotten that EBP is necessary, but not completely sufficient, for the delivery of the highest quality of nursing care. The context of caring that embraces compassion and cultural sensitivity is essential to the provision of safe, competent, and holistic care that meets the health care needs of patients in any setting.

Stephen D. Krau, PhD, RN, CNE
Vanderbilt University Medical Center
School of Nursing
461 21st Avenue South
Nashville, TN 37240, USA

E-mail address:
steve.krau@vanderbilt.edu

REFERENCES

1. Enkin M. Current overviews of research evidence from controlled trials in midwifery obstetrics. J Soc Obstetr Gynecol Can 1992;9:22–33.
2. Available at: http://www.cochrane.org/. Accessed September 16, 2014.
3. Worldviews on Evidence-based Nursing. Available at: http://www.nursingsociety.org/Publications/Pages/WorldviewsRedirect.aspx. Accessed September 16, 2014.
4. Baumann SL. The limitations of evidenced-based practice. Nurs Sci Q 2010;23(3):226–30.

Preface

Evidence-based Nursing: Synthesizing the Best Available Evidence to Translate into Action in Policy and Practice

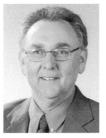

Alan Pearson, AM, RN, ONC, DipNEd, DANS, MSc, PhD,
FCNA, FAAG, FAAN, FRCN
Editor

INTRODUCTION

Evidence-based nursing, although a new term, is a much older concept in both the Eastern and the Western world. Nurses have been talking about, and encouraged to engage in, "research-based practice" for many years. Evidence-based nursing is the same thing as research-based practice in nursing. As more knowledge is generated through research, and as the ability to transmit information via such media as the Internet or direct broadcast increases, all professionals in all fields will come under increasing pressure to show that they are abreast of current knowledge, and that they exhibit this through delivering services that are in line with the most recent and rigorous evidence.

TRANSLATING KNOWLEDGE INTO ACTION IN HEALTH CARE

The rapid development of medical, nursing, and health science over the past fifty years has led to an enormous growth in knowledge. As a result, the expansion in the range of interventions and knowledge available to assist health professionals in their clinical decision-making and to inform service users in making care choices is unprecedented. This burgeoning of knowledge has not, however, necessarily led to an increase in the availability of knowledge to policymakers and clinical practitioners. Many health professionals rely on what they learned in their initial professional training and may be uninformed about current scientific findings. As a result, researchers, policymakers,

Nurs Clin N Am 49 (2014) xiii–xv
http://dx.doi.org/10.1016/j.cnur.2014.09.001
0029-6465/14/$ – see front matter © 2014 Elsevier Inc. All rights reserved.

and political leaders increasingly suggest that the need to constantly translate current knowledge into action at both the policy and the practice levels is poorly addressed.

Knowledge translation is a process derived from the need to ensure that our best knowledge (that is, the best available evidence) is used in practice and involves the ongoing, iterative, and interactive process of translating knowledge from research into clinical practice and policy through ethically sound application and complex interactions between research developers and end users of research.[1–5]

The main principles of knowledge translation are the dissemination of research by researchers, the synthesis of evidence by translational scientists, the utilization of research by policymakers and clinicians, and the implementation of evidence into policy and practice through the transfer of knowledge.[2,6] Knowledge translation strategies therefore require the communication of research findings in ways that influence decision-making, produce effective and collaborative working relationships among all stakeholders (particularly decision-makers and researchers), and ensure that the research is relevant to the intended consumers of that research.[2]

EVIDENCE SYNTHESIS

Evidence synthesis is the evaluation or analysis of research evidence and opinion on a specific topic to aid in decision-making in health care. Although the science of evidence synthesis has developed most rapidly in relation to the meta-analysis of numerical data linked to theories of cause and effect, the further development of theoretical understandings and propositions of the nature of evidence, its role in health care delivery, and the facilitation of improved global health have increased rapidly since 2000.

Pearson and colleagues[7] assert the view that evidence of feasibility, appropriateness, meaningfulness, effectiveness, and economics is legitimate focus for the systematic review process, and that diverse forms of evidence (from experience, opinion, and research that involves numerical and/or textual data) can be appraised, extracted, and synthesized.

The articles appearing in this issue of *Nursing Clinics of North America* examine the role of evidence synthesis in nursing and health care and are written by expert translational scientists from across the world. Three introductory articles overview evidence synthesis and its role in evidence-based health care; methods, issues, and trends in the systematic review of health care evidence; and the development of a robust evidence base for nursing. Subsequent articles explore the impact of systematic reviews on policy and practice in a variety of settings, including perioperative care, pediatrics, rehabilitation and long-term/continuing care, mental health, and public health. The final articles discuss the impact of evidence on health policy and practice and the complexities of translating evidence into policy and practice.

These articles show the importance of synthesizing evidence and translating policy and practice into action in our quest to improve health care and health outcomes.

Alan Pearson, AM, RN, ONC, DipNEd, DANS, MSc, PhD, FCNA, FAAG, FAAN, FRCN
The Joanna Briggs Institute
School of Translation Health Science
Faculty of Health Sciences
The University of Adelaide
Adelaide, Australia

E-mail address:
alan.pearson@adelaide.edu.au

REFERENCES

1. Pyra K. Knowledge translation: a review of the literature. Halifax (NS): Nova Scotia Health Research Foundation; 2003.
2. Bowen S, Martens P. Need to Know Team. Demystifying knowledge translation: learning from the community. J Health Serv Res Policy 2005;10(4):203–11.
3. Lang ES, Wyer PC, Haynes RB. Knowledge translation: closing the evidence-to-practice gap. Ann Emerg Med 2007;49(3):355–63.
4. Mitton C, Adair CE, McKenzie E, et al. Knowledge transfer and exchange: review and synthesis of the literature. Milbank Q 2007;85(4):729–68.
5. Scott NA, Moga C, Barton P, et al, Alberta Ambassador Program Team. Creating clinically relevant knowledge from systematic reviews: the challenges of knowledge translation. J Eval Clin Pract 2007;13(4):681–8.
6. Armstrong R, Waters E, Roberts H, et al. The role and theoretical evolution of knowledge translation and exchange in public health. J Publ Health 2006;28(4):384–9.
7. Pearson A, Wiechula R, Court A, et al. A re-consideration of what constitutes "evidence" in the healthcare professions. Nurs Sci Q 2007;20(1):85–8.

Evidence Synthesis and Its Role in Evidence-Based Health Care

Alan Pearson, AM, RN, ONC, DipNEd, DANS, MSc, PhD, FCNA, FAAG, FAAN, FRCN

KEYWORDS

- Evidence-based health care • Best practice • Nursing

KEY POINTS

- The central role of evidence synthesis (or the systematic review of evidence) in evidence-based health care (EBHC) is often poorly understood by clinicians, academics, and researchers.
- There are numerous examples in the literature of poorly conceived and/or executed systematic reviews and of a lack of awareness of the international standards developed by the international leaders in systematic reviews.
- Most advanced economies—and many low- and middle-income countries—currently identify EBHC as an important component of modern health systems.
- The core of evidence-based practice is the systematic review of the literature on a particular condition, intervention, or issue.

INTRODUCTION

This issue of *Nursing Clinics of North America* focuses on evidence-based health care (EBHC) and the central role of evidence synthesis in this worldwide movement that seeks to improve health outcomes through getting the best available evidence into action in policy and practice. Reflecting the international and cross-disciplinary nature of EGHC, contributing authors come from across the world and from a variety of specialties.

In nursing and all of the health professions, regardless of field or specialty, there is a vast amount of new knowledge created every day. Decision making in health care has

Funding Sources: NHMRC, Centre of Research Excellence Funding.

Conflict of Interest: Previously executive director of the Joanna Briggs Institute and head of the School of Translational Health Science, The University of Adelaide; and director, Cochrane Nursing Care Field, Cochrane Collaboration.

Joanna Briggs Institute, School of Translational Health Science, The University of Adelaide, South Australia 5000, Australia

E-mail address: alan.pearson@adelaide.edu.au

Nurs Clin N Am 49 (2014) 453–460

http://dx.doi.org/10.1016/j.cnur.2014.08.001

0029-6465/14/$ – see front matter © 2014 Elsevier Inc. All rights reserved.

nursing.theclinics.com

changed profoundly over the years for both health professionals and consumers; not only are they expected to make decisions that are based on the best available evidence, but they are also required to review such decisions as new evidence comes to light. The promotion of evidence-based practice, which stems from A.L. Cochrane's work in relation to evidence-based medicine, is gaining momentum in most Westernized countries. Cochrane[1] argued that as resources for health care are limited, they should be used effectively to provide care that has been shown, in valid evaluations, to result in desirable outcomes. In particular, he emphasized the importance of randomized controlled trials in providing reliable information on the effectiveness of medical interventions.

The movement toward EBHC practice thus focuses on the need for all health professionals to use those interventions that are supported by the most up-to-date evidence or knowledge available. The evidence-based approach acknowledges the difficulties faced by busy practitioners in keeping up to date with an ever-growing literature in health care and emphasizes the importance of providing them with condensed information gathered through the systematic review of the international literature on a given topic.

Although there is an international focus on a formalized and multidisciplinary approach to the conduct of systematic reviews and dissemination of evidence-based information, until recently, most activity has been in relation to medicine and evidence-based practice has largely been a synonym for evidence-based medicine. This is changing, however, with nurses and allied health professionals taking increasing interest in establishing an evidence base for their practice, and pursuing strategies to utilize evidence in practice.

THE EMERGENCE OF EVIDENCE-BASED PRACTICE IN THE UNITED STATES AND INTERNATIONALLY

Developments in health care in most Westernized countries over the past 20 plus years have been driven by a desire to minimize unnecessary variability in practice and service delivery and to increase effectiveness.

In the United States, high-cost research and development programs were funded in the early 1990s to develop clinical guidelines generated from systematic reviews, and medical practitioners were encouraged to utilize the synthesised evidence within these guidelines in their daily practice. Thus, until 1995, there was an established strategy in place to review international literature and conduct meta-analyses to generate clinical guidelines based on best available evidence. This was led largely by the Agency for Health Care Policy and Research (AHCPR), which existed between 1989 and 1999, through its funding of Patient Outcomes Research Teams (PORTs). PORTS identified priority health problems and then reviewed and synthesized available research, analyzed practice variations, and developed and disseminated practice guidelines. This program of work came to an end in 1995 largely because of funding cuts and a highly publicized controversy over back surgery. An AHCPR report reviewing research on low back pain concluded that there was no evidence to support spinal fusion surgery. Not surprisingly, the North American Spine Society (NASS) attacked the literature review and the AHCPR practice guideline on acute care of low back pain). With the demise of the AHCPR program, evidence synthesis and clinical guideline development became largely the province of the professional medical associations or colleges. AHCPR became the Agency for Healthcare Research and Quality (AHRQ) and focused, for some years, on other aspects of quality and quality improvement.

However, a resurgence of interest in evidence-based health care began in 2007 when the Institute of Medicine's Round Table published *"Learning What Works Best: The Nation's Need for Evidence on Comparative Effectiveness in Health Care,"*[2] and this was closely followed by the enactment of The American Recovery and Reinvestment Act of 2009 (ARRA). ARRA subsequently took steps toward creating a bigger role for research on comparative effectiveness in the US health system. The AHRQ now has a robust comparative effectiveness portfolio that includes

- The John M. Eisenberg Center for Clinical Decisions and Communications Science, which translates comparative effectiveness reviews and research reports created by AHRQ's Effective Health Care Program into guides and tools for consumers, clinicians, and policymakers
- Evidence-based practice centers that review and synthesize scientific evidence for conditions or technologies that are costly, common, or important to Medicare or Medicaid programs
- The Centers for Education and Research on Therapeutics that conduct research and provide education to advance the optimal use of drugs, biologicals, and medical devices
- The Developing Evidence to Inform Decisions about Effectiveness Network (DECiDE), research-based health organizations that conduct practical studies about the outcomes, comparative clinical effectiveness, safety, and appropriateness of health care items.

Thus, EBHC based on rigorously synthesized evidence is now emerging as an important element of modern health care in the United States.

In the United Kingdom, the British Government directs all major health care provider agencies to develop research and development (R & D) strategies, to establish R & D units, and to promote practices based on best-available evidence. At the same time, the British Government established a number of Centres for Evidence-Based Practice, and these are supported by health research centers such as the Kings Fund for Health Services Development. The strategic development of evidence-based health care in the United Kingdom developed quickly in the early 1990s, with observable benefits. Since the establishment of the Centre for Evidence Based Medicine in Oxford, a linked network of Centres for Evidence Based Practice evolved across the United Kingdom with each center contributing from a specific perspective. In addition, several large-scale initiatives focusing on clinical effectiveness and clinical audit have evolved, as multidisciplinary endeavors and medicine, nursing and allied health professionals are all very much involved in their activities. All of these linked centers bring together focused activities from a range of perspectives to comprehensively contribute to the whole.

In Australia, New Zealand, and Canada, evidence-based health care developed in similar ways as the United Kingdom (although Canada tends to be ahead of the United Kingdom).

Most of the advanced economies (and many low- and middle-income countries) currently identify EBHC as an important component of modern health systems. Evidence-based practice is now almost institutionalized in most industrialized countries, especially in Europe, the United Kingdom, North America, and Australasia. Many of these countries have established centers for EBHC, evidence-based medicine, and evidence-based nursing. For example, there are Cochrane Centres in all of these countries and centers for evidence based nursing in the United Kingdom and North America; additionally, the Joanna Briggs Institute, based in Australia, has 82 collaborating centers throughout Australasia and in Asia, the Americas, Africa, the Middle East, the United Kingdom and Europe.

Globally, there are 3 international, independent, not-for-profit organizations that focus on the sacience of evidence synthesis and translational science.

The Cochrane Collaboration (established in 1993) focuses on the systematic review of randomized controlled trials for specific medical conditions, client groups, or specific health professional interventions. Headquartered in Oxford, United Kingdom, the collaboration links review groups internationally and offers training and support to such groups. Review groups commit to an ongoing process of systematic review in a specific area, and this involves

- Determining the objectives and eligibility criteria for including trials
- Identifying studies that are likely to meet the eligibility criteria
- Tabulating the characteristics and assessing the methodological quality of each study identified
- Excluding studies that do not meet the eligibility criteria
- Compiling the most complete set of data feasible, involving the investigators if possible
- Analyzing the results of eligible studies, using a meta-analysis or statistical synthesis of data if appropriate and possible
- Performing sensitivity analyses if appropriate and possible
- Preparing a structured report of the review that states the aims of the review, describes the materials and methods used, and reports the results

The international Joanna Briggs Institute (established in 1996), with headquarters in Adelaide, South Australia, has over 80 collaborating centers and groups in most Australian states, Asia, Africa, the Middle East, Europe, Canada, the United States, and South America. Given the central role of nursing and allied health in health care delivery, and that the role of nurses and allied health professionals in EBHC has been largely neglected, the Joanna Briggs Institute focuses on the need for an evidence base for nursing and allied health and on assisting health consumers to make informed health decisions. The Joanna Briggs Institute works with researchers, clinicians, and managers to identify those areas in which health professionals most urgently require summarized evidence on which to base their practice. The institute brings together a range of practice-oriented research activities to improve the effectiveness of nursing practice and health care outcomes by

- Conducting systematic reviews and analyses of the research literature
- Collaborating with expert researchers and clinicians to facilitate the development of practice information sheets based on the systematic review of research
- Participating in the dissemination and implementation of best practice information sheets and evaluating their impact on health care practice
- Designing, promoting, and delivering short courses in EBHC for clinicians, researchers, managers, and teachers
- Offering direct fee-for-service consultancies to health service provider agencies to develop customized evidence-based practice training and evidence-based clinical information
- Initiating primary research when indicated by the findings of the systematic review
- Contributing to cost-effective health care through the promotion of EBHC practice
- Planning and organizing regular colloquia to promote knowledge sharing.

The Joanna Briggs Institute seeks to establish working relationships – with other evidence review groups such as the Cochrane Collaboration, the National Health

Service Centre for Reviews and Dissemination (United Kingdom), the National Institute of Clinical Evidence (United Kingdom), the Scottish Intercollegiate Guidelines Network (United Kingdom) and the Agency for Healthcare Research and Quality (United States). The institute is a founding member of the Guidelines International Network (GIN) and of the Nursing International Collaboration in Evidence Based Implementation and Research of Guidelines (NICEBIRG). The institute works alongside these groups and aims to complement their activities to achieve its vision.

The Campbell Collaboration

The Campbell Collaboration (established in 2000) is an international research network headquartered in Norway that produces systematic reviews of the effects of social interventions. It prepares, maintains, and disseminates systematic reviews related to education, crime and justice, social welfare, and international development.

The collaboration operates through 6 coordinating groups that are responsible for the production of Campbell reviews:

- Crime and justice
- Education
- International development
- Methods
- Social welfare and
- Users group

EVIDENCE-BASED HEALTH CARE AND EVIDENCE SYNTHESIS

Simply defined, evidence-based practice is the combination of individual clinical or professional expertise with the best available external evidence to produce practice that is most likely to lead to a positive outcome for a client or patient. Although medicine and nursing are the health care occupations most advanced in the evidence-based practice movement, the ideas and arguments are common to all professionals who work in health care. Sacket and colleagues[3] contend that evidence-based medicine had its philosophic origins in the mid-19th century in Paris. They define it as being "the conscientious, explicit and judicious use of current best evidence in making decisions about the care of individual patients."

These concepts are not without controversy, however. The most controversial issue relates to the current focus on evidence of effectiveness. The dominant approach to the systematic review of evidence favors the meta-analysis of the results of randomized controlled trials (RCTs); indeed, the RCT is conceptualized as the gold standard in evidence of effectiveness, with other quantitative methods ranked as lower in quality in terms of evidence, and the results of interpretive and critical research are not regarded as high-quality evidence. Critics of the prevailing privileging of the RCT and quantitative research cite the argument's inherent critiques of traditional science and the emergence of new paradigms for knowledge. Although the RCT is probably the best approach to generating evidence of effectiveness, nurses, medical practitioners, and other health professionals are concerned with more than cause-and-effect questions, and this is reflected in the wide range of research approaches utilized in the health field to generate knowledge for practice.

Although its proponents would argue that evidence-based practice is not limited to the utilization of the results of traditional research, there has been considerable emphasis on RCTs and meta-analysis, especially in medicine and by the Cochrane Collaboration. This has drawn criticism from those professions that regard qualitative research methods as equally valid forms of research and, thus, generators of legitimate evidence for practice. The result is that qualitative research is generally rendered invisible in systematic reviews. These are a key tool for the evidence-based practice movement. The question here becomes one of what is acceptable research in terms of generating knowledge that amounts to evidence for the purpose of informing practice. There are currently different views on the subject and these generally align with the various positions that characterize the long-standing debate between qualitative and quantitative researchers. This is clearly not an easily resolved argument, but it is vitally important in terms of ascertaining the value of research-generated evidence to health care practices.

Evidence is a complex concept that warrants examination, as it means different things to different people. In its most generic sense, evidence is defined as being the available facts orcircumstances, supporting or otherwise, a belief or proposition or indicating whether a thing is true or valid.[4] There is not a lot of consideration given to the meaning of evidence when attaching this epithet to health care. According to Humphris,[5] the term evidence-based in health care "implies the use and application of research evidence as a basis on which to make health care decisions, as opposed to decisions not based on evidence."

Any indication that a practice is effective, appropriate, meaningful, or feasible—whether derived from experience or expertise or inference or deduction or the results of rigorous inquiry—can be regarded as a form of evidence. The Joanna Briggs Institute regards the results of well-designed research studies grounded in any methodological position as providing more credible evidence than anecdotes or personal opinion; however, when no research evidence exists, expert opinion can be seen to represent the best available evidence.

Pearson and others[6,7] argue for a pluralistic approach when considering what counts as evidence for health care practices, and Evans and Pearson[8] suggest that reviews that include both (or either) qualitative evidence and quantitative evidence are of importance to most practitioners. They go on the suggest, however, that "…optimal methods for reviewing qualitative research are still evolving."

EVIDENCE SYNTHESIS—THE SYSTEMATIC REVIEW

The core of evidence-based practice is the systematic review of the literature on a particular condition, intervention, or issue. The systematic review is essentially a rigorous approach to evidence and involves several steps:

1. The development of a rigorous proposal or protocol. The review protocol provides a predetermined plan to ensure scientific rigor and minimize potential bias. It also allows for periodic updating of the review if necessary. All of the stages of the review are described fully in the protocol, and it is usually subjected to peer review before the review commences.
2. Stating the questions or hypotheses that will be pursued in the review. Questions should be specific regarding the patients, setting, interventions, and outcomes (or, the case of qualitative reviews, phenomena of interest and context) to be investigated.
3. Identifying the criteria that will be used to select the literature. The inclusion criteria should address the participants of the primary studies, the intervention, and the outcomes. In addition to this, it should also specify what research methodologies will be considered for inclusion in the review (eg, randomized controlled trials, clinical trials, case studies, phenomenological studies, and ethnographies).
4. Detailing a strategy that will be used to identify all relevant literature within an agreed time frame. This should include databases and bibliographies that will be searched, and the search terms that will be used.

5. Establishing how the quality of primary studies will be assessed or critically appraised and any exclusion criteria based on quality considerations.
6. Detailing how data will be extracted from the primary research regarding the participants, the intervention, the outcome measures, and the results.
7. Setting out a plan of how the data extracted will be pooled. Statistical analysis (meta analysis) may or may not be used in pooling numerical data, and this will depend on the nature and quality of studies included in the review. Where possible, odds ratio (for categorical outcome data) or standardized mean differences (for continuous data) and their 95% confidence intervals are calculated for each included study. If appropriate with available data, results from comparable groups of studies are then pooled in a statistical meta-analysis using review manager software from the Cochrane Collaboration or the MAStARI software from the Joanna Briggs Institute, which also tests the heterogeneity between the combined results using standard chi-square test.

For qualitative and textual data, qualitative meta-aggregation or meta-ethnography may be used. Where possible, qualitative data are pooled using appropriate software such as the Joanna Briggs Institute's QARI software.

SUMMARY

The central role of evidence synthesis (or the systematic review of evidence) in EBHC is often poorly understood by clinicians, academics, and researchers. There are numerous examples in the literature of poorly conceived and/or executed systematic reviews and of a lack of awareness of the international standards developed by the international leaders in systematic reviews. The Cochrane Collaboration has played a critical global role in developing and refining systematic review methods in relation to evidence of effects and of diagnostic accuracy, and the Joanna Briggs Institute (which follows the methods of Cochrane for effectiveness and diagnostic reviews) has played a similar role in relation to reviews of qualitative, economic, and prevalence-related evidence.

This issue of *Nursing Clinics of North America* examines the state of the art of EBHC in nursing, the processes involved in synthesizing and implementing evidence, and the contribution EBHC has made across a number of specialties.

REFERENCES

1. Cochrane A. 1931-1971: a critical review, with particular reference to the medical profession. In: Medicines for the year 2000. London: Office of Health Economics; 1979. p. 1–11.
2. Institute of Medicine 2011, IOM Roundtable on Evidence-Based Medicine. Learning what works best: the nation's need for evidence on comparative effectiveness in health care: an issue overview. In: Institute of Medicine (US) Roundtable on Value & Science-Driven Health Care, editor. Learning what works: infrastructure required for comparative effectiveness research: workshop summary. Washington, DC: National Academies Press; 2011. Appendix A. Available at: http://www.ncbi.nlm.nih.gov/books/NBK64784/.
3. Sacket DL, Rosenberg W, Gray JA, et al. Evidence-based medicine: what it is and what it isn't. BMJ 1996;312:71–2.
4. Pearsall J, Trumble B. Oxford English reference dictionary. Oxford (United Kingdom): Oxford University Press; 1995. p. 487.

5. Humphris D. Types of evidence. In: Harmer S, Collinson G, editors. Achieving evidence-based practice: a handbook for practitioners. London: Bailliere Tindall; 1999.
6. Pearson A. Evidence-based nursing: quality through research. In: Nay R, Garratt S, editors. Nursing older people: issues and innovations. Sydney (Australia): Maclennan & Petty; 1999. p. 338–52.
7. Pearson A, Wiechula R, Court A, et al. A re-consideration of what constitutes "evidence" in the healthcare professions. Nurs Sci Q 2007;20(1):85–8.
8. Evans D, Pearson A. Systematic reviews: gatekeepers of nursing knowledge. J Clin Nurs 2001;10:593–9.

The Systematic Review of Health Care Evidence

Methods, Issues, and Trends

Fiona Bath-Hextall, PhD

KEYWORDS

- Systematic reviews • Synthesis • Health care evidence • Methods

KEY POINTS

- The systematic review is a key component to the evidence based health care cycle.
- Systematic reviews bring together large amounts of information that can help support individual patient decision, inform guidelines, policy and can inform primary research.
- There are two main types of systematic reviews: qualitative and quantitative. The basic steps for each type of systematic review are the same; however, differences occur in the tools used to appraise the included studies and the method of synthesis.

WHAT IS A SYSTEMATIC REVIEW?

The systematic review is a key component to the evidence-based health care cycle, (**Fig. 1**).

A systematic review, as the name implies, is undertaken systematically. It is a structured body of work undertaken by a group of people according to an explicit methodology that is reproducible and answers a clearly focused question. Systematic reviews can be used to resolve uncertainty when primary research, reviews, and editorials disagree.

HOW DO THEY DIFFER FROM OTHER REVIEWS?

A word of caution: systematic reviews are not the same as literature reviews. A literature review done by one expert in the field might draw very different conclusions to another literature review done by another expert in the field; literature reviews are not reproducible (**Table 1**). Guidelines for the better reporting of systematic reviews

Disclosures: none.
Conflicts of interest: none.
Centre for Evidence Based Healthcare, School of Health Sciences, Queen's Medical Centre, University of Nottingham, Nottingham NG7 2UH, UK
E-mail address: Fiona.bath-hextall@nottingham.ac.uk

Nurs Clin N Am 49 (2014) 461–473
http://dx.doi.org/10.1016/j.cnur.2014.08.002

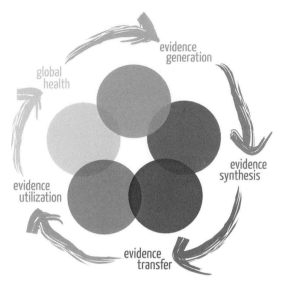

Fig. 1. Evidence based healthcare cycle.

were established in 1999 by the Quality of Reporting of Meta-analysis initiative[1] but are now superseded by the PRISMA (Preferred Reporting Items for Systematic Reviews and Meta-Analyse) statement for reporting systematic reviews and meta-analyses.[2] If you are ever in doubt as to whether a review has been undertaken systematically, then these guidelines serve as a useful checklist for the reporting of systematic reviews.

WHAT ARE SYSTEMATIC REVIEWS USED FOR?

Health care professionals are overwhelmed with unmanageable amounts of information. Systematic reviews bring together large amounts of information that can be easily digested that can help support individual patient decisions, inform guidelines and policy, and inform and direct research. Clinical studies may have insufficient power to detect modest but important effects; however, a meta-analysis can improve

Table 1
Differences between literature reviews and systematic reviews

	Literature Review	Systematic Review
Framing the question	Often broad	Well structured
Searching for the evidence	Not usually specified (not reproducible)	Clear and reproducible
Methodological quality of the evidence	Variable	Rigorous critical appraisal
Synthesis	Often qualitative summary	May be qualitative (with/without a meta-synthesis) or quantitative (with/without a meta-analysis) depending on the question
Interpreting the findings	May be biased	Usually evidence based

the precision of these measures of effect by statistically combining the data from multiple studies and calculating a new single measure of effect, called the *pooled result*.

DIFFERENT TYPES OF SYSTEMATIC REVIEWS

There are 2 main types of systematic reviews: qualitative and quantitative. The basic steps for each are the same; however, differences occur in the data extraction and synthesis. Although both quantitative and qualitative systematic reviews have their strengths, any review that focuses exclusively on one form of evidence presents only half the picture and will, therefore, have limited applicability in many contexts. Three general frameworks have been proposed for the undertaking of mixed-method systematic reviews.[3] The segregated methodologies maintain a clear distinction between quantitative and qualitative evidence, and individual synthesis is conducted before the final mixed-method synthesis. Integrated methodologies directly bypass separate quantitative and qualitative syntheses and instead combine both forms of data into a single mixed-method synthesis. A primary condition for the development of an integrated mixed-method systematic review is that both qualitative and quantitative data are similar enough to be combined into a single synthesis. Contingent methodologies involve 2 or more syntheses conducted sequentially based on results from the previous synthesis.[4] At present, there is no consensus as to how these mixed-method reviews should be undertaken; however, the Joanna Briggs Institute (JBI) thinks that mixed-method reviews are more inclusive and can produce a synthesis of evidence that is more accessible to a wider audience. JBI has adopted the segregated approach to mixed-method synthesis. This mixed-method synthesis uses a Bayesian approach to translate the findings of the initial quantitative synthesis into qualitative themes and pooling these with the findings of the initial qualitative synthesis.[4]

More recently, systematic reviews of existing reviews are being undertaken to compare and contrast published reviews and to provide an overall examination of a body of information that is available for a given topic.[5] These reviews go by various names (*umbrella reviews, overviews of reviews,* or *reviews of reviews*) and are a means of summarizing the results of multiple systematic reviews covering different interventions for the same clinical condition. Overviews could be a useful resource for policy makers in developing clinical practice guidelines and decision support systems. These reviews extract the results as reported in the component systematic reviews and do not aim to repeat or update the literature searches, eligibility assessment, bias assessment, or statistical synthesis from the reviews that are summarized.

Standard meta-analyses are an effective tool in evidence-based health care, but one of their drawbacks is that they can only compare 2 alternative treatments at any one time. So if no studies exist that directly compare 2 interventions, then it is not possible to estimate their relative efficacy. Multiple treatments meta-analysis (MTM) is a new emerging methodology that uses a meta-analysis technique that allows the incorporation of evidence from both direct and indirect comparisons from a network of trials of different interventions to estimate summary treatment effects.[6–8] This methodology can be referred to as *MTM, mixed treatment comparisons*, or *network meta-analysis.*

WHERE TO FIND REVIEWS

Some useful Web sites for locating systematic reviews can be seen in **Box 1**. The Cochrane Database of Systematic Review is mostly concerned with quantitative

---

Box 1
Web sites for finding systematic reviews

The Cochrane Library: http://www.thecochranelibrary.com/view/0/index.html

Centre for Reviews and Dissemination: http://www.york.ac.uk/inst/crd/

The Joanna Briggs Institute Library: http://joannabriggslibrary.org/

Evidence-Based Nursing: http://ebn.bmj.com/

Turning Research Into Practice Database: http://www.tripdatabase.com/

The Campbell Library: http://www.campbellcollaboration.org/lib/

---

reviews, overviews of reviews, and methodology reviews; however, last year, Cochrane published its first qualitative systematic review.[9] The JBI Database of Systematic Reviews and Implementation Reports includes both quantitative and qualitative reviews and, more recently, umbrella reviews. The Campbell Collaboration is an international research network that produces systematic reviews of the effects of social interventions on policy and services.

UNDERTAKING A SYSTEMATIC REVIEW

The steps for undertaking a systematic review are shown in **Box 2**.

The protocol of a systematic review can be thought of as a recipe. It specifies a predetermined plan as to how the review will be undertaken. It is crucial to establish the method of a protocol before the review is done, so as to avoid biases. A good protocol will have clearly stated objectives including a clearly focused question, clear methods for the identification of the studies of their assessment, and how they will be summarized. The methods described should be rigorous and clearly defined and should have repeatability; that is, someone else should be able to replicate the methods.

Step 1: Framing the Question

Developing a structured question is the first step in undertaking a systematic review and should not be underestimated; it is not easy and takes a lot of practice but, once mastered, is an invaluable skill for both clinicians and researchers alike. It is crucial that you take your time over this step, as the review question underpins all aspects of the review methodology. A well-focused question helps with the search strategy, provides guidance for inclusion of studies, and guides the data extraction and synthesis of the results. There are many different types of research questions, and different types of questions will need to be answered by different types of study designs (**Table 2**).

Box 2
Steps in conducting systematic reviews

1. Asking a clearly focused question
2. Searching for the evidence
3. Looking at the quality of the evidence
4. Summarizing/synthesizing the evidence
5. Interpreting the findings

Table 2
Different types of study for different types of questions

Question	Study Type
Questions about intervention	RCT
Etiology: What factors cause these problems? Risks: What risk factors predict disease? Prognosis: What happens with this disease over time? Diagnosis: If the test is positive, what happens to the client?	Cohort
Risks: What risk factors predict disease? Prognosis: What happens with this disease over time?	Case control
Frequency: How common is the outcome (disease)? Etiology: What risk factors are associated with these outcomes?	Cross-sectional
Phenomena of interest: Why do patients...? How do carers feel about...?	Qualitative research (interviews, focus groups, participant observation)

Abbreviation: RCT, randomized controlled trial.

It has been proposed that a well-built question contains 3 or 4 components.[10–12] A range of mnemonics are available to help with the structuring of review questions; the most common for quantitative reviews is PICO, which stands for *P*articipants, *I*ntervention/exposure, *C*omparison, and *O*utcome. However, PICO is less helpful if you are trying to frame a qualitative question. JBI offers an alternative to PICO that can be used to frame qualitative questions (**Box 3**). Further alternative mnemonics to help with framing qualitative questions have been proposed, such as *SPICE* (Setting, Perspective, Intervention, Comparison, Evaluation)[13] and *SPIDER* (Sample, Phenomenon of Interest, Design, Evaluation and Research type).[14] For diagnostic test accuracy reviews, the mnemonic *PIRATE* (*P*opulation, *I*ndex test, *R*eference test, *A*ccuracy methods, *T*est cutoff points, *E*xpected test use) has been proposed (**Box 4**).

Step 2: Searching for the Evidence

Once an appropriate question has been formulated, then we can proceed to find the best available evidence to answer the question. Searching for evidence is a real skill and needs to be learned. Because this is an evolving field, it is often advisable to seek help from a library search specialist.

The aim of a good search strategy is to maximize the chances of finding as many studies as possible, both published and unpublished. This strategy involves searching as widely as possible using a whole range of sources.

Numerous electronic databases are available; however, only the ones relevant to the question should be used. Each database has its own characteristics; although you might use similar search terms for diseases or interventions or clinical trials,

Box 3
Framing a qualitative question

Population characteristics

Phenomena of interest

Context

> **Box 4**
> **The mnemonic *PIRATE* can be used to help frame a diagnostic accuracy question**
>
> *P*opulation/participants
>
> *I*ndex test: What are the tests under evaluation in the review?
>
> *R*eference test: To what test are the index tests going to be compared with (ie, what is the best test currently available)?
>
> *A*ccuracy methods: How will accuracy be measured (sensitivity, specificity, likelihood ratios, and predictive values)?
>
> *T*est cutoff point: How will the data be dichotomized? What constitutes positive and negative results should be clearly defined for both the index and reference test.
>
> *E*xpected test use: What is the anticipated role of the index test?

they will be indexed and displayed differently in each database. The key to an effective search is using the appropriate keywords. When searching for the evidence, you will need to think of all of the different ways to describe your research area/topic and compile a list of synonyms that describe your topic. Keyword or natural language searching will retrieve the exact terms that you key into a database search box. The database will search in the title and abstract fields of the articles to find research papers whereby the exact same terms have been used by authors. Some databases also produce a list of subject headings, sometimes referred to as *descriptors*, to overcome the problems associated with different spellings or different interpretations of a subject. So articles on the same topic should be indexed using the same descriptor. These terms are controlled terms, which are added to every research article in a database to aid consistency. Some examples include Medical Subject Headings (MeSH), which are used in Medline, and the Cumulative Index to Nursing and Allied Health Literature subject headings, which are used with the Cumulative Index to Nursing and Allied Health database. Subject headings can help to focus searches and find more relevant articles.

The structure of a search strategy should be based on the framed question, as in the case of the following PICO: Is alcohol gel more effective than soap and water for preventing [methicillin-resistant *Staphylococcus aureus*] MRSA/Clostridium dificile in hospitalized patients. The Boolean terms *AND* and *OR* are used to combine search terms (**Table 3**).

The search strategy for each database needs to be clearly recorded together with the date the search was undertaken. This point is particularly pertinent because new records have constantly been added to new databases and methods of indexing are constantly being developed.

In addition to searching for published material, there should also be searches for gray literature; ongoing studies; and, in some cases, there may be a need for hand searching of journals.

Expert opinion may also be important, especially for rare conditions when little evidence may be available.

Search filters can be very useful as they are designed to retrieve records of research using a specific study design. Filters are usually published for a specific database interface, and **Box 5** gives some useful Web pages for locating search filters.

Some of the problems with searching include publication and language bias.[15] Publication bias is when positive results tend to be published more frequently than negative results in journals,[16] and language bias is when positive results are more likely to be published in English.[17]

Table 3
Framed question used to help with search strategy

Column Terms Combined with	Patients AND	Intervention AND	Comparison AND	Outcomes AND
OR	1. Hospitalized patients (keyword)	1. Alcohol gels (keyword)	1. Soap (keyword)	1. C diff (keyword)
OR	2. Hospitalized patients (keyword)	2. Alcohol hand rubs (keyword)	2. Soaps (keyword)	2. Clostridium difficile (keyword)
OR	3. Hospitalization (keyword)	3. Alcohol-based hand rubs (keyword)	3. Hand disinfection (MeSH)	3. MRSA (keyword)
OR	4. Hospitalization (keyword)	4. Gels (MeSH)	4. Hand hygiene (MeSH)	4. Clostridium difficile (MeSH)
OR	5. Patient hospitalized (keyword)	5. Alcohols (MeSH)		5. Methicillin-resistant *Staphylococcus aureus* (MeSH)
OR	6. Patients in hospital (keyword)	6. Antiinfective agents (MeSH)		
OR	7. Inpatients (MeSH)	7. Patients in hospital (MeSH)		
	8. Combine 1–7 using *OR*	8. Combine 1–7 using *OR*	5. Combine 1–4 using *OR*	6. Combine 1–5 using *OR*

The last step is to combine lines 8 + 8 + 5 + 6 with *AND*.
Patient, hospitalized patients; *Intervention,* alcohol gel; *Comparison,* soap and water; *Outcome,* reduction in spread of MRSA/C diff.
Keywords and MeSH headings using PICO (US and UK spellings).

After the search has been completed, studies need to be selected for inclusion or exclusion in the review. Two reviewers should independently look at the titles and abstracts of all the studies retrieved from the search and include only those that meet the predefined inclusion criteria. The next stage is to obtain the full text for those studies included in the first screening and then read the full text of each study to see if they meet the inclusion criteria. It is very important that a record is kept of this process, and it should be detailed in a search flow diagram (**Fig. 2**).

Box 5
Useful Web addresses for locating search filters

Scottish Intercollegiate Guideline network Search filters: http://www.sign.ac.uk/methodology/filters.html

Inter TASC Information Specialists' Sub-Group: https://sites.google.com/a/york.ac.uk/issg-search-filters-resource/issg

Clinical evidence: http://clinicalevidence.bmj.com/x/set/static/ebm/learn/665076.html

The University of Nottingham Centre of Evidence Based Healthcare: a Collaborating Centre of the Joanna Briggs Institute: http://www.nottingham.ac.uk/research/groups/cebhc/resources.aspx

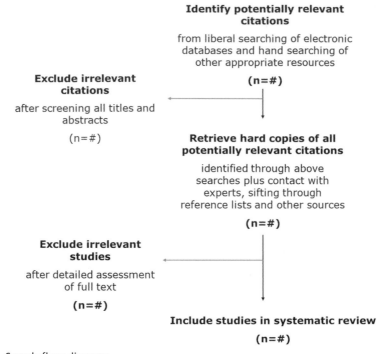

Fig. 2. Search flow diagram.

Step 3: Looking at the Quality of the Evidence

Evidence can come from many different types of studies, and unfortunately not all studies are done well.

Critical appraisal is an integral process in evidence-based practice and looks at the extent to which a study is free from methodological biases. Appraising the quality of studies allows the exploration of how differences in quality might explain differences in the study results and will guide the interpretation of the findings and their value to practice. The criteria for looking at the quality of quantitative and qualitative studies differ; therefore, it is essential to use the appropriate tool. There are numerous appraisal tools available to assess the quality of primary studies. The International Centre of Allied Health Evidence has an excellent Web page that links directly to the Web sites where the appraisal tools were developed (www.unisa.edu.au/cahe/).[18]

Two reviewers should independently look at the methodological quality of each study, and any disagreements should be resolved by a third reviewer.

Step 4: Synthesizing the Evidence

Before the synthesis stage, data extraction needs to be undertaken; because every systematic review question is different, this is normally done using a tailor-made data extraction sheet.

Quantitative systematic reviews use a characteristic set of methods for analyzing data, called *meta-analysis*. Meta-analysis is "a statistical analysis that combines or integrates the results of several independent clinical trials considered by the analyst to be combinable"[19–21] and then calculates a new single measure of effect (pooled result or summary statistical). Sometimes it is not appropriate to undertake a meta-analysis, especially if the studies identified have exposures and outcomes that have been measured in different ways.

The most commonly used measure of effect for categorical data is the odds ratio (OR), or the relative risk (RR), also called *risk ratio*. Other measures of effect are risk reduction (percentage difference in the risk of having an event between the 2 groups) and number needed to treat, which tells you how many patients would need to be treated with the new treatment in order to prevent the event occurring in one patient. The most commonly used measure of effect for numerical data is called the *mean difference*, calculated by subtracting means of the data in the 2 treatment groups. Meta-analysis gives different weights to each of the studies, with larger studies given relatively more weight than the smaller studies. Forest plots are used to present the results from a meta-analysis (**Table 4**). The center of the diamond at the bottom of the plot represents the pooled measure of effect, and the width of the diamond relates to the confidence intervals. Heterogeneity is the degree to which the results from the studies vary, and a meta-analysis should only be performed when heterogeneity is not a problem. Heterogeneity can be assessed visually by looking at the forest plot and checking if the results from each study lie within the 95% confidence intervals of the pooled results, or a statistical test called I^2 can be used to assess the level of heterogeneity between the results of the studies (see **Table 4**).[22] The value for I^2 ranges from 0% to 100%. An I^2 of 50% indicates that 50% of the total variation in the meta-analysis is caused by heterogeneity. An I^2 value between 85% and 100% means that the studies are too different and not comparable.

Two main methods are used to calculate the summary statistical. The *fixed effect method* is when a weighted average of the RR is calculated using data from all of the different studies, where the weight is proportional to the size of the study, and so the larger the study the more influence it will have on the pooled RR. This method assumes that all of the available studies were trying to estimate a true value that is the same for all of them. This method can be used when the estimates visually vary but their confidence intervals more or less overlap. This validity of using the fixed effect method can be assessed using the I^2 statistical; where a fixed effect model is appropriate when I^2 is between 0% and 30% to 40%. If I^2 has a value between 40% and 85%, then a more appropriate method is the *random effect method*, which accounts for some of the heterogeneity between studies.

Table 4
Forest plot

Study or Subgroup	Intervention A Events	Total	Placebo Events	Total	Weight	Risk Ratio M-H, Random, 95% CI	Risk Ratio M-H, Random, 95% CI
Reference 1	4	24	10	11	7.1%	0.18 [0.07, 0.46]	
Reference 2	23	96	26	32	21.1%	0.29 [0.20, 0.44]	
Reference 3	70	364	349	360	31.0%	0.20 [0.16, 0.25]	
Reference 4	17	84	77	82	19.5%	0.22 [0.14, 0.33]	
Reference 5	21	68	21	24	21.4%	0.35 [0.24, 0.52]	
Total (95% CI)		636		509	100.0%	0.25 [0.19, 0.32]	
Total events	135		483				
Heterogeneity: Tau² = 0.05; Chi² = 9.22, df = 4 (P = .06); I² = 57%							0.01 0.1 1 10 100
Test for overall effect: Z = 10.19 (P<.00001)							Favors treatment A Favors placebo

Abbreviation: CI, confidence interval.

Studies of diagnostic accuracy are conducted to determine the accuracy of a test used to diagnose conditions. The accuracy is plotted against a standard reference test. A diagnostic test is any test used in making a diagnosis based on the presenting signs and symptoms or monitoring the progression of a disease or condition.[23] For systematic reviews of diagnostic test accuracy, the outcome measures reported are summary measures of test accuracy: sensitivity, specificity, likelihood ratios (the probability that a particular result will occur in a patient with the disease, compared with the probability that someone without the disease would have the same results), and receiver operator characteristic (ROC) curve information (plots of sensitivity and specificity). ROC curves are used to determine the overall diagnostic accuracy of a test. The *Cochrane Handbook of Systematic Reviews of Diagnostic Test Accuracy*[24] highlights how the meta-analysis of diagnostic test accuracy differs from the meta-analysis of interventions and also covers the main aspects of data analysis.[25]

The synthesis of economic data does not follow the same pattern as other reviews. There are 3 options for the synthesis of economic data. The results can be presented as a narrative summary, sorted into tables by comparisons or outcomes, or they can be summarized using a permutation matrix.[26] The choice of synthesis will depend on the quality and quantity of the evidence identified. The JBI has developed a permutation matrix called the *Analysis of Cost, Technology, and Utilization Assessment and Review Instrument*. The matrix uses a dominance rating whereby each intervention is placed in a position on a grid depending on whether it is preferred over its comparator. The matrix has 3 possible outcomes, which are determined by the reviewer's rating of the economic evidence and presented visually. These ratings can be for either the intervention or the comparison: (1) The process is less expensive or more clinically effective (strong dominance). (2) Interventions are comparable or equal for cost or clinical effectiveness. There is weak dominance that supports either clinical effectiveness or cost-effectiveness but not both. (3) The intervention is less expensive. Nondominance exists when the intervention of interest is less effective or more costly.

For qualitative systematic reviews, there are various approaches to meta-synthesis. They vary in the degree of interpretation involved with the approaches, such as meta-ethnography, which is highly interpretive, and meta-aggregation, which is less interpretive and more integrative.[27] For meta-aggregation, the reviewer does not reinterpret the primary research findings from each paper but works with the interpretations that primary researchers made in the first place. This approach involves extraction of findings from the included papers, categorizing the findings, and then aggregating these categories to develop synthesized findings (**Figs. 3** and **4**). This approach is favored by JBI. In contrast to meta-aggregation, meta-ethnography is a form of interpretive synthesis in which the researcher tries to generate new meanings rather than deduce existing meanings.[28] The findings are not aggregated but are analyzed and reinterpreted to generate in the form of explanatory, midlevel, or substantive theory. The goal is not explicitly to inform or provide recommendations for practice, but it aims to develop conceptual models of understanding.[29]

Step 5: Interpreting the Findings

The ultimate purpose of a systematic review is to facilitate health care decision making. The idea is to present information and aid interpretation rather than to offer recommendations. The discussions and conclusions should help people understand the implication of the evidence in relation to practical decision and apply the result to their specific situation.

The validity of the findings will depend on the strengths and weaknesses of the review. The following will need to be considered: Are the searches adequate? Is there a

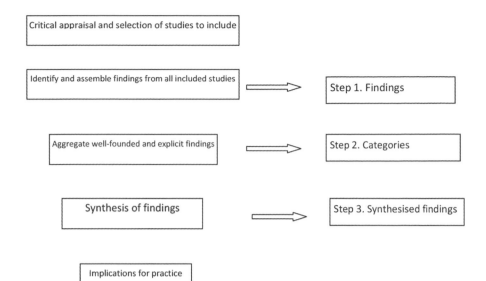

Fig. 3. Steps in meta-aggregation.

risk of publication and related biases? Is the quality of the included studies good enough? Are the observed effects clinically significant and not just statistically significant?

Publication bias is when you are more likely to identify published studies that have found interesting (usually positive) results rather than less interesting (usually negative) ones. The funnel plot can be used to explore publication bias by looking at the magnitude of the OR against the precision of the study.[17] If no publication bias exists, then the funnel plot will be approximately symmetric. The effects of publication bias can be

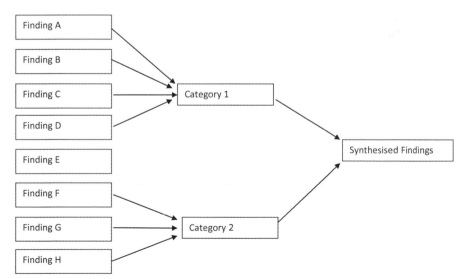

Fig. 4. Relationship between findings, categories, and synthesized findings.

reduced by making sure that the review of published literature is as thorough as possible and by additional hand searching through references quoted by each paper to make sure everything is found.

Over the years, many different systems have been used to grade the quality (level) of evidence and the strength of recommendations, which has meant that the same evidence and recommendation could be graded differently according to the system used at the time.

The Grade of Recommendations, Assessment, Development, and Evaluation (GRADE) Working Group has developed a system for grading the quality of evidence and strength of recommendations.[30] For the purpose of the systematic review, the GRADE approach defines the quality of a body of evidence as the extent to which one can be confident that an estimate of effect or association is close to the quantity of specific interest. The quality of a body of evidence involves consideration of the within-study risk of bias (methodological quality), directness of evidence, heterogeneity, precision of effect estimates, and risk of publication bias. The GRADE system involves an assessment of the quality of a body of evidence for each individual outcome.[25]

The Cochrane collaboration has adopted the GRADE system for evaluating the quality of evidence for outcomes reported in systematic reviews. More recently, the GRADE approach has also been adopted by JBI for reviews addressing questions of effect/therapy and a modified GRADE approach to the summary of finding for other reviews other than effect/therapy.

REFERENCES

1. QUOROM (Quality of Reporting of Meta-analyses) guidelines. These guidelines were first published in 1999, providing guidance to ensure the proper reporting of systematic reviews. Available at: http://www.biomedcentral.com/content/supplementary/1471-2261-10-24-s1.pdf. Accessed September 28, 2014.
2. Liberati A, Altman DG, Tetzlaff J, et al. The PRISMA statement for reporting systematic reviews and meta-analyses of studies that evaluate healthcare interventions: explanation and elaboration. BMJ 2009;339:b2700.
3. Sandelowski M, Volis CI, Barosso J. Defining and designing mixed research synthesis studies. Res Sch 2006;13(1):29.
4. JBI Reviewers' Manual 2014 Edition. Available at: http://joannabriggs.org/assets/docs/sumari/ReviewersManual-2014.pdf. Accessed September 28, 2014.
5. Hartling L, Chisholm A, Thomson D, et al. A descriptive analysis of overviews of reviews published between 2000 and 2011. PLoS One 2012. http://dx.doi.org/10.1371/journal.pone.0049667.
6. Cipriani A, Barbui C, Rizzo C, et al. What is a multiple treatments meta-analysis? Epidemiol Psychiatr Sci 2012;21:151–3. http://dx.doi.org/10.1017/S2045796011000837.
7. Caldwell DM, Ades AE, Higgins JP. Simultaneous comparison of multiple treatments: combining direct and indirect evidence. BMJ 2005;331:897.
8. Salanti G, Higgins JP, Ades AE, et al. Evaluation of networks of randomized trials. Stat Methods Med Res 2008;17(3):279–301.
9. Glenton C, Colvin CJ, Carlsen B, et al. Barriers and facilitators to the implementation of lay health workers programmes to improve access to maternal and child health: qualitative evidence synthesis. Cochrane Database Syst Rev 2013;(10):CD010414. http://dx.doi.org/10.1002/14651858.CD010414.pub2.

10. Richardson W, Wilson M, Nishikawa J, et al. The well-built clinical question: a key to evidence-based decisions [editorial]. ACP J Club 1995;123:A12–13.
11. Sackett DL, Rosenberg W, Taylor DW, et al. Clinical determinants of the decision to treat primary hypertension. Clin Res 1977;24:648.
12. Flemming K. Asking answerable questions. Evid Based Nurs 1998;1(2):36–7.
13. Booth A. Clear and present questions: formulating questions for evidence based practice. Libr Hi Tech 2006;24(3):355–68.
14. Cooke A, Smith D, Booth A. Beyond PICO: the SPIDER tool for qualitative evidence synthesis. Qual Health Res 2012;22(2):1435–43.
15. Dickersin K, Chan S, Chalmers TC, et al. Publication bias and clinical trials. Control Clin Trials 2002;8:343–53.
16. Bruce N, Pope D, Stanistreet D. Quantitative methods for health research: a practical interactive guide to epidemiology and statistics. London: Wiley; 2008.
17. Egger M, Zellweger-Zahner T, Schneider M, et al. Language bias in randomized controlled trials published in English and German. Lancet 1997;350(9074):326–9.
18. Links to critical appraisal tools. Available at: http://www.unisa.edu.au/Research/Sansom-Institute-for-Health-Research/Research-at-the-Sansom/Research-Concentrations/Allied-Health-Evidence/Resources/CAT/#RCT.
19. Huque MF. Experiences with meta-analysis in NDA submissions. Proceedings of the Biopharmceutical Section of the American Statistical Association 1988;2:28–33.
20. Egger M, Smith GD. Meta-analysis: potential and promise. BMJ 1997;315:1371–4.
21. Cook DJ, Mulrow CD, Haynes RB. Systematic reviews: synthesis of best evidence for clinical decisions. Ann Intern Med 1997,126(5).376–80.
22. Higgins JP, Thompson SG, Deeks JJ, et al. Measuring inconsistency in meta-analysis. BMJ 2003;327:557–60.
23. Macaskill P, Gatsonis C, Deeks JJ, et al. Chapter 10: Analysying and Presenting Results. In: Deeks JJ, Bossuyt PM, Gatsonis C, editors. Cochrane Handbook for Systematic Reviews of Diagnostic Test Accuracy Version 0.9.0. The Cochrane Collaboration, 2010. Available at: http://srdta.cochrane.org/. Accessed September 28, 2014.
24. Macaskill P, Gatsonis C, Deeks JJ, et al. Chapter 10: analysing and presenting results. In: Deeks JJ, Bossuyt PM, Gatsonis C, editors. Cochrane handbook for systematic reviews of diagnostic test accuracy version 1.0. The Cochrane Collaboration; 2010. Available at: http://srdta.cochrane.org/.
25. Schünemann HJ, Oxman AD, Vist GE, et al. Chapter 12: interpreting results and drawing conclusions. In: Higgins JP, Green S, editors. Cochrane handbook for systematic reviews of interventions version 5.1.0. The Cochrane Collaboration; 2011. Available at: www.cochrane-handbook.org.
26. Nixon J, Khan KS, Kleijnen J. Summarising economic evaluations in systematic reviews: a new approach. BMJ 2001;322:1596–8.
27. Finfgeld-Connett D. Generalisability and transferability of meta-synthesis research findings. J Adv Nurs 2010;66(2):246–54.
28. Noblit GW, Hare R. Meta-ethnography: synthesizing qualitative studies. Newbury Park (CA): Sage; 1988.
29. Holly C, Salmond SW, Saimbert MK, editors. Comprehensive systematic review of advanced nursing practice. New York: Springer Publishing Company, LLC; 2011.
30. Guyatt GH, Oxman AD, Vist G, et al, GRADE Working Group. Rating quality of evidence and strength of recommendations GRADE: an emerging consensus on rating quality of evidence and strength of recommendations. BMJ 2008;336:924–6.

Developing a Robust Evidence Base for Nursing

CrossMark

Lisa Hopp, PhD, RN, FAAN

KEYWORDS

- Systematic review • Joanna Briggs Institute • Cochrane Collaboration • PRISMA
- Best available evidence

KEY POINTS

- Systematic reviews are ideal best evidence because they are based on an exhaustive search and transparent rigorous methods.
- Systematic reviews are inconsistently identified in bibliographic databases and knowledge users need critically appraise them using standard criteria.
- More nurses need to be prepared to conduct systematic reviews using internationally developed standard practices.

Over the last 2 decades, nursing care has begun to transform toward clinical decisions informed by the best available evidence and clinical expertise, and made by engaging patients to illuminate and incorporate their circumstances, preferences, and values. However, the transformation is in its early days. It is a steep challenge to live up to the "best available evidence" element in the definition of evidence-based practice. This paper will address initiatives in the United States and internationally to systematically develop an evidence base for nursing care and critically evaluate progress and strategies to enhance it through systematic reviews focused on nursing care.

ROBUST EVIDENCE BASE

The Oxford dictionary defines robust as "strong, health and vigorous." Synonyms include "sturdy in construction," "strong," and "able to withstand or overcome adverse conditions."[1] This definition indicates that robust evidence can withstand criticism, is defensible and of sufficient magnitude (ie, vigorous) to make a difference. Currently, a wide assortment of evidence sources within the discipline of nursing and among other disciplines exists to inform nursing practice, but not all of them are robust. Knowledge users need to ask fundamental questions of these sources of evidence to judge whether or not the source should inform their decisions. Most importantly they need to ask, "How does the source achieve the qualification of being

Disclosure: None.
College of Nursing, Purdue University Calumet, 2200 169th Street, Hammond, IN 46323, USA
E-mail address: ljhopp@purduecal.edu

Nurs Clin N Am 49 (2014) 475–484
http://dx.doi.org/10.1016/j.cnur.2014.08.003   **nursing.theclinics.com**

best available?" Whether the source is a system of evidence, a practice guideline, a systematic review, or a single study, it can only be defensible if it can be judged for how it is the best of available evidence.

Increasingly, vendors and publishers are marketing sources as being evidence based. They need to be able to respond to the users who ask, "How does your knowledge source represent the best available evidence?" If they respond with answers like "there are references," "we have an expert editorial board," or "many organizations use our system," but do not support how they developed the system, guideline, and so on, to meet the standard of best available, it cannot be judged as robust or even defended as "evidence based."

Implications of "Best Available Evidence"

Definitions of evidence-based health care consistently include reference to "best evidence"[2] and publications about searching include finding the "best available evidence."[3,4] Both words, best and available, have important implications for finding and selecting evidence for making clinical decisions. To determine the best evidence, clinicians need to have methods to judge the quality of the evidence using criteria to benchmark it relative to ideal evidence. Finding available evidence implies that the search process is comprehensive and exhaustive, but that ideal evidence may not be available. Then clinicians need to use other sources of evidence to inform decisions while understanding that the evidence may be more vulnerable to biases.

Many authors and organizations have proposed hierarchies of evidence quality and other hierarchies that qualify the strength of the recommendations that stem from the evidence. These hierarchies assist knowledge users in weighing the strength of the evidence and their confidence in the information gained from it. Many hierarchies relate only to questions of effect, so the study designs logically relate to those that would appropriately address comparative effectiveness, like randomized controlled trials. Knowledge users need other hierarchy systems for other kinds of questions like those of diagnosis, prognosis, etiology, risk, and meaning of experience. For example, it is not logical or appropriate to study the meaning of a lived experience using a quantitative design like a randomized controlled trial. Therefore, for questions like, "What is the experience of dyspnea in patients in an acute exacerbation of heart failure?", need an appropriate hierarchy where the strongest evidence uncovers that experience through a systematic review of qualitative evidence. On the other hand, questions of effectiveness cannot be answered with qualitative evidence; rather, a systematic review of well-conducted, randomized, controlled trials is the ideal source of evidence.

Systematic reviews rise to the top of evidence hierarchies because they are designed to systematically search all available studies (published, unpublished, all languages), and critically appraise and synthesize the world's evidence on a particular question.[5,6] They must be transparent in their methods to be accountable and explicit.[7] A systematic review of quantitative evidence may or may not include a metaanalysis (statistical pooling) of data extracted from the included studies. Although metaanalyses provide parameters to judge the precision of the pooled effect, they do not necessarily ensure additional rigor of a systematic review and are just 1 component of a systematic review of quantitative evidence. Systematic reviews of qualitative evidence use the same steps as a quantitative systematic review and produce metaaggregations and synthetic statements. These statements can guide practice and understanding of patients' experiences through the metasynthesis of findings from qualitative studies.[8]

Systematic review methods have developed over the past 2 decades and represent international consensus about how to properly conduct a rigorous systematic review.

International organizations like the Cochrane and Campbell Collaborations, the Joanna Briggs Institute (JBI) and Collaboration continuously examine and improve the methodologies. Other types of literature reviews exist, such as realist reviews, state of the science/art reviews, rapid reviews, and systematized reviews.[9] These reviews have different purposes, scopes, and may not be as exhaustive in their search processes or synthesize findings in reproducible ways. Generally, they have not undergone the same methodologic development as a systematic review and are not found in evidence hierarchies. Thus, they are not meant to inform clinical decisions in the same manner as a systematic review or even individual sources of primary research.

When someone has made the claim that a source is evidence based, the knowledge user expects that the source reflects the best available evidence and that it can live up to its definition. If a source lacks transparency in how it represents both the best and the available evidence, the claim of being evidence based is suspect. Any so-called evidence-based information needs to supply the search strategy so the knowledge user can assess how exhaustively and logically the authors hunted for the available evidence. Authors of the evidence-based resource need to divulge the methods of appraisal and if they have ranked the quality of the evidence or recommendations, they need to define the hierarchical system.

TRENDS IN PUBLICATION OF SYSTEMATIC REVIEWS RELEVANT TO NURSING
Finding Systematic Reviews

No single database of systematic reviews relevant to nursing practice and care exists. Rather, systematic reviews can be found in many places, including bibliographic databases; specialized online libraries like the Cochrane, Campbell, and JBI Libraries; government websites that house systematic reviews like the Agency for Healthcare Quality and Research (AHRQ); and other society and academic websites (**Table 1**). Some online resources are registries of systematic reviews published elsewhere and indexed by other sources but they provide summaries, appraisal and commentary about the review. The University of York's Center for Reviews and Dissemination[10] is one such database where they provide access to 30,000 quality-assessed systematic reviews, 15,000 economic evaluations, and 12,000 health technology assessments. Using the search term "nurs*" in any field of the Center for Reviews and Dissemination

Table 1
Counts of systematic reviews in databases, February 2004 to January 2014

Database	No. of Systematic Reviews
PubMed	28,216
Cochrane	8343
CINAHL	31,275
JBI	301
AHRQ	143

PubMed is the National Library of Medicine's database; search: "systematic review" in title.
  Cochrane is the Cochrane Database of Systematic Reviews; search: all systematic reviews.
  CINAHL is the Cumulative Index of Nursing and Allied Health Literature; search: systematic review publication type limiter.
  JBI is the Joanna Briggs Institute Library; search: all systematic reviews over the data range.
  AHRQ is the Agency for Health Research and Quality; search: list of systematic review reports published by evidence-based practice centers.

database netted 3985 systematic reviews. However, this registry does not capture all reviews, although they update it every day.[11] Other groups assemble evidence from the published literature, summarize it briefly, and assess or comment on the evidence quality and clinical relevance. One such resource is McMaster University Health Information Research Unit's Best Evidence for Nursing Plus service. They have assembled evidence as far back as 2002, including 3761 matches for "systematic review."[12] Users can find some full-text articles through a link to PubMed. McMaster University offers similar services in other disciplines that may be useful for nursing, including for health systems, public health, and rehabilitation.[13]

Overview of Published Systematic Reviews Relevant to Nursing Care

Challenges exist in trying to capture how many systematic reviews exist that are relevant to nursing practice and to describe what areas of practice are covered well and where the gaps exist. Databases identify systematic reviews in different ways; some exist only in separate libraries, whereas others are indexed redundantly among several databases. Some bibliographic platforms and databases use systematic review in their publication type limiter and others do not. Even when the limiter is available, the rules used to apply the limiter are not transparent and the definition may include reviews that would not qualify as a systematic review. The Cumulative Index to Nursing and Allied Health Literature (CINAHL) via EBSCOhost states that a systematic review:

Indicates a research process in which a concept is identified and the research which has studied it is analyzed and evaluated. The results of this research are synthesized to present the current state of knowledge regarding the concept. Includes integrated or integrative reviews.[14]

Another approach is to search for "systematic review" in the title. Reviewers often use this phrase in the title of the publication so they can be found by limiting the search to the title field. When comparing the 2 search techniques in CINAHL over the same 20-year period, using the publication type limiter of systematic review returned 22,281 more hits than using "systematic review" in title.

We examined a small random sample of 20 of 3700 full-text publications identified by the systematic review limiter to understand what types of articles are tagged as systematic reviews in the database. Five of the 20 were Cochrane systematic reviews and they are indexed appropriately as systematic reviews. Although none of these included "systematic review" in the title, all of them included the usual characteristics of a systematic review, including an a priori published protocol, transparency in search methods and results, dual reviewers using inclusion criteria, risk of bias assessment, and clear methods of analysis and synthesis. The other 15 were very heterogeneous in the clarity of the question and transparency in methods. One was a casual literature review with no methodology, one was a letter with some methods, one was a concept analysis, and two were reviews of basic pharmacologic or biological science. Eight of the 15 included "systematic review" in the title and had some but not all of the characteristics of a systematic review. For example, none identified that an a priori protocol guided the review, and some lacked assessment of risks of bias or using dual reviewers to improve reliability of appraisal and extraction methods. Even this small sample reveals that knowledge users must be critical consumers and evaluate the rigor of the methods, particularly in a general database like CINAHL.

It was not possible to duplicate the same type of search in Medline because no limiter for systematic review exists for the database. However, when we searched PubMed from February 1994 through January 2014 using "systematic review" AND "nurs*" in the title, 1742 records resulted. In this search, 5 of the top 10 journals were nursing focused journals, including *Journal of Advanced Nursing* (n = 98), *Journal of Clinical Nursing* (n = 55), *International Journal of Nursing Studies* (n = 48), *International Journal of Evidence Based Healthcare* (n = 39), and *Worldview on Evidence Based Nursing* (n = 20). Interestingly, duplicating the same strategy in CINAHL netted fewer matches than in Medline.

Although indexing may be imperfect, CINAHL and the JBI Library (not yet indexed in CINAHL) are most focused on publishing systematic reviews relevant to nursing, so they are examined more closely herein to determine gaps.

Bibliographic Trends in Nursing: Cumulative Index to Nursing and Allied Health Literature 1994 to 2014

To assess the number of systematic reviews indexed through the CINAHL database, a search was conducted in 5-year segments from February 1994 to January 2014 using both the publication type limiter, systematic review, with no key word search and the phrase "systematic review" in the title field. Overall, using the limiter, 31,275 publications were found, whereas 10,468 were found when "systematic review" was in the title. Despite the difficulties in identifying systematic reviews, it is clear that their number has increased dramatically in the last decade, increasing more than 9-fold when comparing citations 10 years before and after 2004 by using the systematic review limiter (**Fig. 1**).

Because CINAHL includes integrative reviews in their limiter, combining "integrative review" in the title with the systematic review publication type limiter yielded 519 of 31,275 matches for "integrative review." The methodology for an integrative review may or may not be similar to a systematic review; its methodology has not undergone the same development and consensus building by international experts as systematic reviews. Integrative reviews tend to be syntheses of studies of varying designs, but

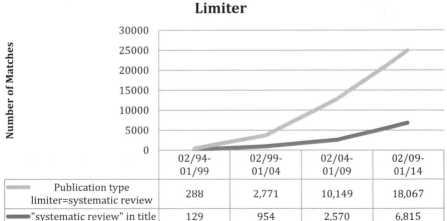

Fig. 1. Trends in systematic review publication from February 1994 to January 2014 using 2 search techniques in the Cumulative Index of Nursing and Allied Health Literature (CINAHL) database.

they may lack elements of the standard methodology of systematic reviews, such as dual reviewers, standardized appraisal tools, an analysis of risk of bias, complete transparency in methods, or an a priori published review protocol.

In the future, registries may ease how knowledge users find and identify legitimate systematic review protocols and the final report. Systematic reviews published by the 3 major international organizations (Cochrane, Campbell, and JBI Library) and, increasingly, public funding agencies, require that peer reviewers approve the protocol that guides the review before the reviewers commence the project. These protocols are published and indexed in their respective libraries. In addition, these organizations and their authors participate in the University of York's Centers for Reviews and Dissemination international prospective register of protocols called PROSPERO.[10] Reviewers search the database before embarking on a systematic review to limit redundancies. In addition, methodologic transparency is enhanced when knowledge users can compare how the reviewer planned and subsequently carried out the review. These registries and libraries of systematic reviews simplify searching and enhance rigor through peer review and methodologic consistency.

Geographic and gender distribution
Despite its lack of precision, but because of its feasibility, we searched using the publication limiter to determine the geographic distribution of systematic review authors from February 1994 to January 2014. Europe (n = 14,048), the United Kingdom and Ireland (n = 13,156), and the United States (n = 12,854) were the top 3 producers, followed by continental Europe (n = 2104), and Australia and New Zealand (n = 1619). Mexico and Central/South America (n = 775), Canada (n = 586), and Asia (n = 233) also had substantial contributions. Gender was specifically identified in a portion of the findings. Females (n = 6002) were more commonly the target population than males (n = 3547).

Publishers of systematic reviews
During the same 20-year period, the majority of systematic reviews indexed in CINAHL were published in journals focused more on medical practice rather than nursing practice (see **Table 1**). By far, the Cochrane Database of Systematic Reviews yielded the most reviews (n = 5445). Although many of these reviews are of interest to nursing care, a much greater portion relate directly to decisions relevant to physician practice. Only 2 journals specifically focused on nursing practice ranked in the top 11 publishers of systematic reviews: The *Journal of Advanced Nursing* published 371 and the *Journal of Clinical Nursing* published 250.

Subject major headings
Major subject headings in the CINAHL provide some insight into the focus of systematic reviews over the last 2 decades. The top subject heading was the rather broad category of treatment outcomes (n = 1136) followed by stroke (n = 684), depression (n = 527), and quality of life (n = 467; **Fig. 2**).

Nursing practice foci
Because the major headings are broad, we undertook a second approach to try to capture what areas of specialty practice are best informed by systematic review. Using CINAHL's categories of nursing disciplines,[15] we searched the database using the systematic review publication type limiter and the date range from February 2004 to January 2014. In each case, we joined each appropriately truncated key word with "AND nurs*" to try to capture reviews relevant to nursing and the area of nursing care. For example, to find systematic reviews relevant to cancer nursing care, we searched

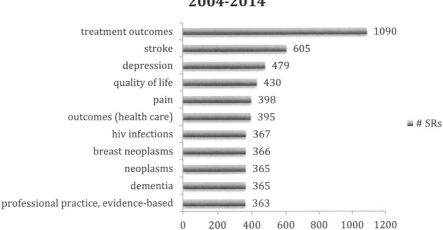

Fig. 2. Major headings in Cumulative Index of Nursing and Allied Health Literature (CINAHL) systematic reviews (SR) from 2004 to 2014.

(oncolog* AND nurse) OR (cancer AND nurs*). Oncology/cancer, critical care/emergency/trauma, perioperative/surgical nursing, and psychiatric nursing netted the top 4 categories, accounting for nearly half of the total searched (1578/3235; **Fig. 3**). We also searched on elements of the nursing process using interv* AND nurs*, assess* AND nurs*, and diagnos* AND nurs*. Nursing intervention netted 1313 systematic reviews, assessment 864, and diagnosis 476.

Bibliographic Trends in Nursing: Joanna Briggs Institute Library (1998 to 2014)

The JBI Library has been publishing systematic reviews since 1998, but before 2004 only 16 were in the library and 285 were published between 2004 and 2014.[16] The JBI is an international research unit housed at the University of Adelaide and linked with 70 international entities contributing to the evidence-based practice endeavor and the JBI Library. Many of these centers and groups focus on evidence synthesis so they train others in the methodology and produce systematic reviews for the library. All of the systematic reviews use a common, standardized approach to the conduct of the review including peer review and publication of a priori protocols, standard appraisal, and data extraction tools and analysis and reporting software. Their approach is parallel to the Cochrane Collaboration, except that they conduct both quantitative and qualitative systematic reviews.[16] The JBI Library is the only international organization with focused methodologic and software development of qualitative metasynthesis.

The library is organized into 16 specialty nodes, such as aged care, burns care, cancer care, mental health, midwifery, rehabilitation, and wound care. Unlike its companion organizations of the Cochrane and Campbell collaborations, most of the reviews are directly relevant to nursing care. The most fully populated specialty node is the aged care node, with 55 systematic reviews followed by chronic disease at 42 and pediatrics at 32. The other nodes all have 17 to 26 reviews each. The burns care and wound healing and management nodes are very small with only 2 and 3 reviews, respectively (**Fig. 4**).

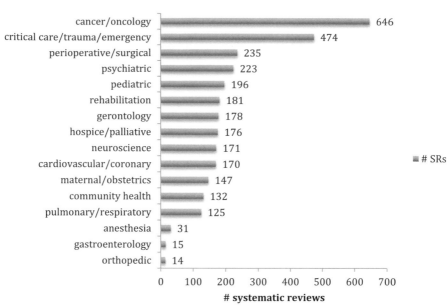

Fig. 3. CINAHL Nursing Foci from 2004-2014. Search used systematic review publication type limiter; appropriate truncation of each key term combined with the truncated term, nurs*, in any field.

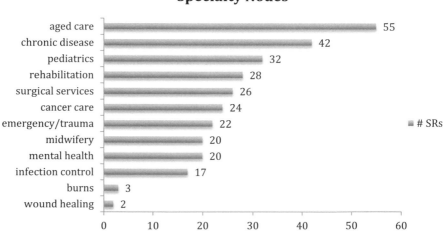

Fig. 4. Joanna Briggs Institute (JBI) Library distribution of systematic reviews in specialty nodes from 2004 to 2014.

Gaps in Systematic Review Literature for Nursing Care

Despite the inherent difficulties in describing the body of systematic reviews, there are some conclusions that can be made regarding gaps and needs for the future. Cancer and oncology nursing seems to have the greatest number of systematic reviews to inform practice as evidenced by searches of CINAHL and the JBI Library. Aged care, gerontology and chronic disease topics are also making good progress. The least developed areas in these 2 nursing databases include gastroenterologic nursing and anesthesia nursing. That being said, no area of nursing practice is overstudied.

Building a Robust Evidence Base for Nursing in the Future

Searching CINAHL using publication type limiters or title searching revealed too much variability in how systematic reviews are identified. Knowledge users need a more standard approach that enables them to easily and authentically identify systematic reviews. Systematic reviewers need to use methodologies that represent the most rigorous approaches developed through international debate and consensus building. Too many systematic reviews, particularly in the nonspecialty libraries, lack critical quality elements. This threatens their credibility. Missing quality elements include refereed, publically available protocols, clear transparent methods that include inclusion criteria, search strategies and results, appraisal and risk of bias assessment, using at least 2 reviewers, and approaches to extraction, coding and synthesis. International standards for reporting systematic reviews exist, but they are not universally adopted. The PRISMA statement includes 27 items on a checklist that addresses each part of a systematic review.[17] The statement has been reprinted in a number of journals, but none of them are nursing journals.[18]

Systematic review is a legitimate form of research and schools of nursing need to routinely teach the methodology so that more reviews can be developed to inform nursing practice. Practicing nurses and nurse scientists who wish to conduct systematic reviews can seek training from expert groups like Cochrane and the JBI centers.

SUMMARY

Systematic reviews provide robust evidence for nursing practice because of the exhaustiveness of search, the critical appraisal methods to determine the risks of bias and synthesis methods that pool evidence to increase the power of statistical estimates or credibility of aggregated metasynthesis of qualitative findings. More consistency in publication standards will enhance the rigor of available evidence and allow nursing to live up to the promise of best, available evidence.

REFERENCES

1. Oxford Dictionaries. Definition of "robust". Available at: http://www.oxforddictionaries.com/us/definition/american_english/robust?q=robust. Accessed March 1, 2014.
2. Sackett DL, Rosenberg WC, Muir JA, et al. Evidence based medicine: what it is and isn't. BMJ 1996;312:71–2.
3. Rosenberg W, Donald A. Evidence based medicine: an approach to clinical problem-solving. BMJ 1995;310:1122–6.
4. GRADE Working Group. Grading quality of evidence and strength of recommendations. BMJ 2004;328:1490–4.
5. Straus SE, Glasziou P, Richardson WS, et al. Evidence-based medicine: how to practice and teach it. Edinburgh (Scotland): Churchill Livingston Elsevier; 2011.

6. Pearson A, Weeks S, Stern C. Translation science and the JBI model of evidence-based healthcare. Philadelphia: Lippincott Williams and Wilkins; 2011.

7. Gough D, Oliver S, Thomas J. An introduction to systematic reviews. Los Angeles (CA): Sage; 2012.

8. Pearson A, Robertson-Malt S, Rittenmeyer L. Synthesizing qualitative evidence. Philadelphia: Lippincott Williams and Wilkins; 2011.

9. Grant MJ, Booth A. A typology of reviews: An analysis of 14 review types and associated methodologies. Health Info Libr J 2009;26:91–108.

10. University of York Centres for Reviews and Dissemination. About CRD. 2012. Available at: http://www.york.ac.uk/inst/crd/about_us.htm. Accessed March 1, 2014.

11. University of York Centres for Reviews and Dissemination. Welcome to PROSPERO International prospective register of protocols. 2013. Available at: http://www.crd.york.ac.uk/PROSPERO/. Accessed March 1, 2014.

12. Best Evidence for Nursing Plus. Welcome. 2014. Available at: http://plus.mcmaster.ca/np/Default.aspx. Accessed March 1, 2014.

13. McMaster Health Information Unit. McMaster Plus. Available at: http://hiru.mcmaster.ca/hiru/HIRU_McMaster_PLUS_projects.aspx. Accessed March 1, 2014.

14. EBSCOhost CINAHL Support Center. CINAHL via EBSCOhost! Available at: http://www.ebscohost.com/resources/cinahl-plus-with-full-text/lma/document-types.htm. Accessed March 1, 2014.

15. EBSCOhost CINAHL Support Center. Nursing disciplines covered. Available at: http://www.ebscohost.com/resources/cinahl-plus-with-full-text/lma/subject-headings.htm. Accessed March 1, 2014.

16. Joanna Briggs Institute. Joanna Briggs Institute library. Available at: http://joannabriggslibrary.org/. Accessed March 1, 2014.

17. Moher D, Liberati A, Tetzlaff J, et al. Preferred reporting items for systematic reviews and meta-analyses: the PRISMA statement. PLoS Med 2009;6(7):1–6.

18. PRISMA. The PRISMA statement. Available at: http://www.prisma-statement.org/usage.htm. Accessed March 1, 2014.

Evidence in Perioperative Care

Dru Riddle, DNP, CRNA[a],*, Daphne Stannard, PhD, RN, CNS[b],*

KEYWORDS

- Perioperative • Evidence-based practice • Systematic review

KEY POINTS

- Perioperative care is comprised of three care areas: preoperative, intraoperative, and postoperative care.
- Given the vulnerable status of the perioperative patient, coupled with the complex nature of these areas, EBP and clinical decision-making must be rooted in high-quality evidence for safe and effective patient and family care.
- EBP is comprised of three critical elements: patient and family preferences, clinical expertise, and best available evidence.
- Systematic reviews provide the highest quality of evidence.

INTRODUCTION

Perioperative care encompasses a wide array of disciplines, providers, and patient interactions and is typically divided into three care areas: (1) preoperative, (2) intraoperative, and (3) postoperative care. Peri means "around" in Greek, and perioperative areas wrap themselves around the patient's operative experience to safely care for and guide the patient and family through the entire perioperative continuum.[1] Although these care areas may not be geographically dispersed (because some patients are prepared and recovered in the same area where the procedure occurred), they are considered three distinct phases of care, whereby different clinical objectives are met and unique skills are required for each phase. However, because phase of care is frequently associated with phase I and II recovery,[2] the term "care area" is used throughout this article to refer to preoperative, intraoperative, and postoperative care.

Disclosure: None.
[a] TCU Center of Evidence Based Practice and Research: A Collaborating Center of the Joanna Briggs Institute, School of Nurse Anesthesia, Texas Christian University, TCU Box 298626, Fort Worth, TX 76108, USA; [b] Institute for Nursing Excellence, UCSF Centre for Evidence-Based Patient and Family Care: An Affiliate Centre if the Joanna Briggs Institute, Surgical Services Node, Joanna Briggs Institute, University of California San Francisco Medical Center, 2233 Post Street, Suite 201, Box 1834, San Francisco, CA 94115, USA
* Corresponding authors.
E-mail addresses: d.riddle@tcu.edu; Daphne.stannard@ucsfmedctr.org

A hallmark of perioperative care is interdisciplinary collaboration, because there are front-line clinicians who directly interface with the patient and family, but also scores of staff who help to support the safe movement of the patient and family through the care trajectory. The disciplines of surgery, anesthesia, nursing, pharmacy, respiratory therapy, rehabilitative specialists, laboratory, and radiology technicians, among many other allied health members, all intersect in the perioperative arena.

In addition to the direct care clinicians and support staff, numerous consultants and specialists also have a role in providing perioperative care to patients undergoing surgery and anesthesia. Use of consultants is seen throughout all phases of perioperative care: preoperatively for risk stratification and optimization; intraoperatively for diagnostic and therapeutic consultation; and postoperatively for patient management, rehabilitation, and long-term planning. Finally, the importance of patients' families cannot be overlooked as an important source of support, especially preoperatively and postoperatively. As a system, the perioperative environment is the gestalt of a complex system in which multiple pieces work in tandem to accomplish a common goal.[3]

That most patients move across three care areas during the course of their surgical procedure speaks to this complexity, along with all of the moving clinicians, equipment, and handoff communications. For that reason, the number one driving force in perioperative care is patient safety. The activities of all individuals providing care, making decisions, and ultimately interacting with the patient and family need to be based on the premise that reduction of risk and optimizing outcomes are the overarching goals.[4]

Despite the complexity in perioperative areas, evidence-based practice (or EBP) is no different than EBP in other areas. Some evidence is more rigorous and higher on the evidence pyramid compared with other types of evidence. Systematic reviews are widely held to be the highest form of evidence and when conducted well, a systematic review identifies, critically appraises, and synthesizes the best available evidence for a specific clinical question to improve patient and family care and to guide decision-making and policy.[5] The use of systematic reviews as evidence in informing health care decisions is not a novel concept; however, the frequency of its use has increased tremendously in the past 5 years.[6] A properly executed systematic review contains the following defining features:

- A well-defined question
- An a priori protocol guiding the review
- Clear and specific inclusion and exclusion criteria
- Transparent and reproducible search strategy
- Assessment of methodologic quality for included studies
- Data assimilation strategies congruent with methodology
- Clear and robust recommendations for practice

There are several public and private sector organizations that produce systematic reviews, including the Cochrane Collaboration, Campbell Collaboration, and the Joanna Briggs Institute (JBI). The Cochrane Collaboration produces systematic reviews of health care interventions based on quantitative evidence, and the Campbell Collaboration produces systematic reviews on the effects of social interventions based on quantitative evidence. JBI, however, has a more pluralistic view of evidence and produces systematic reviews of health-related practices and interventions based on quantitative and qualitative evidence.

JBI was founded in 1996 and is an international not-for-profit, research and development arm of the School of Translational Science based within the Faculty of Health

Sciences at the University of Adelaide, South Australia. JBI collaborates with more than 70 entities across the world. JBI and its collaborating entities promote and support the synthesis, transfer, and use of evidence through identifying feasible, appropriate, meaningful, and effective health care practices to assist in the improvement of health care outcomes globally. It is worth noting that JBI has more than 15 nodes (with more under development) that are comprised of clinicians and researchers working within a specialty area (eg, surgical services). The members of the node review and help to coordinate the further development of node resources. The Surgical Services Node is an active node comprised of clinicians from around the world interested in advancing perioperative and perianesthesia care to improve patient and family outcomes and experiences. A list of systematic reviews filtered by the Surgical Services Node is listed in **Table 1**.

SYSTEMATIC REVIEWS IN PERIOPERATIVE CARE

In this field, systematic reviews often focus on one perioperative care area. Although much overlap exists between the various care areas, evidence to inform practice is commonly divided among preoperative, intraoperative, and postoperative care. Additionally, evidence informing perioperative care tends to be discipline specific, with systematic reviews focusing on nursing, medicine, surgery, and anesthesia practice as examples.

Perioperative systematic reviews, much like systematic reviews in other disciplines of health care, focus on improving patient and family outcomes. Because of the complexity of perioperative care, systematic reviews in this area often focus on risk reduction and improved outcomes. Stratifying risk throughout all phases of perioperative care has been the recent focus of systematic reviews. In the following sections, selected systematic reviews that focus on the different components of perioperative care are highlighted.

PREOPERATIVE CARE

Westerdahl and Tenling[7] completed a systematic review focusing on the effectiveness of preoperative physical therapy on reducing the risk of developing postoperative atelectasis and pneumonia in patients undergoing elective cardiac surgery. The authors concluded that preoperative physical therapy decreased the incidence of atelectasis and pneumonia and decreased hospital length of stay.[7] Although this systematic review focused on the preoperative period, the impact of the intervention is seen in the postoperative period. Additionally, this systematic review highlights the interaction between multiple disciplines providing care in the perioperative period.

Bradt and coworkers[8] published another systematic review specific to the preoperative period. The focus of this review was to determine the effectiveness of listening to music preoperatively on preoperative anxiety. The authors concluded that there was a significant reduction in preoperative anxiety scores for those patients that were exposed to music in the preoperative period compared with those in the control group.[8] In this review, all studies measured anxiety using the State-Trait Anxiety Index, with anxiety reduction reported as 5.72 units less in the music group compared with the control group.[8] As with the previous review, Bradt and coworkers[8] highlight the dynamic nature of the care components within the perioperative arena. Although often temporally removed and physically distant, an effective intervention performed preoperatively (in this case, listening to music) can reap significant benefits once the patient reaches the surgical unit postoperatively.

Table 1
Perioperative systematic reviews in the JBI database of systematic reviews and implementation reports filtered by surgical node (as of March 8, 2014)

Number	Citation
1	Aguilera-Martinez R, Ramis-Ortega E, Carratala-Munuera C, et al. Effectiveness of continuous enteral nutrition versus intermittent enteral nutrition in intensive care patients: a systematic review. JBI Database of Systematic Reviews and Implementation Reports 2014;12(1):281–317.
2	Chair SY, Fernandez R, Liu M, et al. The clinical effectiveness of length of bed rest for patients recovering from trans-femoral diagnostic cardiac catheterization. JBI Database of Systematic Reviews and Implementation Reports 2008;9(47):1971–98.
3	Chan TW, Mackey S, Hegney D. Patients' experiences towards the donation of their residual biological samples and the impact of these experiences on the type of consent given for secondary use: a systematic review. JBI Database of Systematic Reviews and Implementation Reports 2011;9(42):1714–81.
4	Charnock Y. The nursing management of chest drains. JBI Database of Systematic Reviews and Implementation Reports 2001.
5	Conroy T. The prevention and management of complications associated with established percutaneous gastrostomy tubes in adults: a systematic review. JBI Database of Systematic Reviews and Implementation Reports 2009;7(1):1–37.
6	Crowe L, Chang A, Fraser J, et al. Systematic review of the effectiveness of nursing interventions in reducing or relieving post-operative pain. JBI Database of Systematic Reviews and Implementation Reports 2008;6(4):165–224.
7	Evans D. Music as an intervention for hospital patients. JBI Database of Systematic Reviews and Implementation Reports 2001.
8	Fernandez R, Griffiths R, Murie P. Comparison of late night and early morning removal of short-term urethral catheters. JBI Database of Systematic Reviews and Implementation Reports 2003.
9	Fernandez R, Griffiths R, Ussia C. Effectiveness of solutions, techniques, and pressure in wound cleansing. JBI Database of Systematic Reviews and Implementation Reports 2004.
10	Froessler B, Tufanaru C, Cyna A, et al. Preoperative anemia management with intravenous iron: a systematic review. JBI Database of Systematic Reviews and Implementation Reports 2013;10(11):157–89.
11	Gollaher T, Baker K. Administration of propofol of non-mechanically ventilated patients in non-critical care areas by anesthesia providers and non-anaesthesia trained healthcare providers: a systematic review. JBI Database of Systematic Reviews and Implementation Reports 2012;10(46):2944–97.
12	Hewitt V, Watts R. The effectiveness of non-invasive complementary therapies in reducing postoperative nausea and vomiting following abdominal laparoscopic surgery in women: a systematic review. JBI Database of Systematic Reviews and Implementation Reports 2009;7(19):850–907.
13	Hines S, Chang A, Ramis MA, et al. Effectiveness of nurse-led preoperative assessment services for elective surgery: a systematic review. JBI Database of Systematic Reviews and Implementation Reports 2010;8(15):621–60.
14	Hoon L, Hong-Gu H, Mackey S. Parental involvement in their school-aged children's post-operative pain management in the hospital setting: a comprehensive systematic review. JBI Database of Systematic Reviews and Implementation Reports 2011;9(28):1193–225.
15	Jones S, Merrill A. Effectiveness of intravenous acetaminophen for pain management in orthopedic surgery patients: a systematic review. JBI Database of Systematic Reviews and Implementation Reports 2012;10(37):2490–513.

(continued on next page)

	Table 1 (*continued*)
Number	**Citation**
16	Lockwood C, Conroy-Hiller T, Page T. Vital signs. JBI Database of Systematic Reviews and Implementation Reports 2004.
17	Martin S, Jordan Z, Carney A. The effect of early oral feeding compared to standard oral feeding following total laryngectomy: a systematic review. JBI Database of Systematic Reviews and Implementation Reports 2013;11(11):140–82.
18	McLiesh P, Wiechula R. Identifying and reducing the incidence of post discharge venous thromboembolism (VTE) in orthopedic patients: a systematic review. JBI Database of Systematic Reviews and Implementation Reports 2012;10(41):2658–710.
19	Merrill A, Jones S. Effectiveness of surgical weight loss on the remission of type 2 diabetes mellitus: a systematic review. JBI Database of Systematic Reviews and Implementation Reports 2012;10(36):2465–89.
20	Moola S, Lockwood C. The effectiveness of strategies for the management and/or prevention of hypothermia within the adult perioperative environment: a systematic review. JBI Database of Systematic Reviews and Implementation Reports 2010;8(19):752–92.
21	Mu PF, Wang KW, Chen YC, et al. A systematic review of the experiences of adult ventilator-dependent patients. JBI Database of Systematic Reviews and Implementation Reports 2010;8(8):343–81.
22	Ng C, Bialocerkowski A, Hinman R. Effectiveness of arthroscopic versus open surgical stabilization for the management of traumatic anterior glenohumeral instability. JBI Database of Systematic Reviews and Implementation Reports 2007;5(4):230–78.
23	Nur L, Creedy D. A comprehensive systematic review of factors influencing women's birthing preferences. JBI Database of Systematic Reviews and Implementation Reports 2012;10(4):232–306.
24	Phillips N, Haesler E, Street M, et al. Post-anaesthetic discharge scoring criteria: a systematic review. JBI Database of Systematic Reviews and Implementation Reports 2011;9(41):1679–713.
25	Picheansathian W. Effectiveness of alcohol-based solutions for hand hygiene. JBI Database of Systematic Reviews and Implementation Reports 2004.
26	Robertson-Malt S, Barbary M. Prophylactic steroids for paediatric open-heart surgery: a systematic review. JBI Database of Systematic Reviews and Implementation Reports 2008;6(5):225–33.
27	Siah R, Childs C. A systematic review of surgical infection scoring systems using in surgical patients. JBI Database of Systematic Reviews and Implementation Reports 2011;9(60):2627–83.
28	Sng Q, Taylor B, Zhu L, et al. Children's experiences of their postoperative pain management: a qualitative systematic review. JBI Database of Systematic Reviews and Implementation Reports 2013;11(4):1–66.
29	Stern C, Lockwood C. Knowledge retention from preoperative patient information. JBI Database of Systematic Reviews and Implementation Reports 2005.
30	Thompson L. Suctioning adults with an artificial airway. JBI Database of Systematic Reviews and Implementation Reports 2000.
31	Vlayen A, Verelst S, Bekkering G, et al. Exploring unplanned ICU admissions: a systematic review. JBI Database of Systematic Reviews and Implementation Reports 2011;9(25):925–59.
32	Walker M, Kralik D, Porritt K. Fasciotomy wounds associated with acute compartment syndrome: a systematic review of effective treatment. JBI Database of Systematic Reviews and Implementation Reports 2014;12(1):101–75.
33	Wiechula R. Post harvest management of split thickness skin graft donor sites. JBI Database of Systematic Reviews and Implementation Reports 2001.

INTRAOPERATIVE CARE

First published in 2008 and then updated in 2013, Modolo and colleagues[9] report on the differences between intravenous and inhaled anesthesia during one-lung ventilation surgeries.[10] The authors aimed to determine if there was a difference in postoperative outcomes when intravenous or inhaled anesthesia was used during surgery for maintenance of anesthesia. The authors found no difference in outcomes based on the type of anesthesia used during the surgical procedure.[9] The choice of the anesthetic technique during one-lung ventilation surgeries had no determination on the postoperative outcomes extant in the literature. This systematic review highlights the importance of publishing nonsignificant findings. Because different anesthesia techniques all have economic implications to the health care system, even nonsignificant findings from systematic reviews, such as Modolo and colleagues, can have an important clinical impact.

Occasionally, there are multiple systematic reviews that cover the same topic. In these situations, it may be appropriate to perform an overview of systematic reviews (also known as an umbrella review), whereby the results of each systematic review are combined together to produce a robust practice recommendation. One such umbrella review combined nine Cochrane systematic reviews to determine the best anesthetic technique for prevention of postoperative mortality and major morbidity after surgery.[11] Based on the outcomes of each individual review, the authors concluded that central neuraxial blockade with either spinal or epidural anesthesia may reduce the zero- to 30-day mortality for patients undergoing surgery when that surgery possesses an intermediate-to-high cardiac risk level.[11] The authors concluded that the risk of mortality following intermediate-to-high cardiac risk level surgery is 29% less when spinal or epidural anesthesia is used compared with general anesthesia.[11]

POSTOPERATIVE CARE

In a recent systematic review, Riddle and Nugent[12] focused on the effectiveness of intraoperative brain activity monitoring on postanesthesia care unit (PACU) length of stay. The authors concluded that a statistically nonsignificant 3.47-minute reduction in PACU length of stay can be realized if intraoperative brain activity monitoring is used to help guide the delivery of anesthesia. Although statistically insignificant, any reduction in PACU length of stay may have clinical significance, especially in crowded and underbedded PACUs. In a 20-bed PACU, reducing length of stay for each patient by 3 minutes has the cumulative effect of reducing PACU usage by 1 full hour.

The postoperative time period is often loosely used: it can be defined as immediately after anesthesia and the surgical procedure to long-term postprocedure. A systematic review highlighting the effectiveness of continuous passive movement following total knee arthroplasty is an example of long-term outcomes in the postoperative period.[13] In 2014 the authors reported an update to a 2003 and 2010 systematic review on the same topic. It was determined that the use of continuous passive movement machines following total knee arthroplasty does not have clinically important effects on active knee range of motion, pain, function, or quality of life. The authors conclude that the routine use of continuous passive movement machines in the postoperative period following total knee arthroplasty should not be routinely recommended.[13] Using evidence such as this to guide practice is incumbent on all practitioners, because unnecessary equipment delays early mobilization and drives up health care costs.

CASE STUDY

One of the most common complaints reported by patients in the perioperative period is the inability to eat or drink anything after midnight on the day preceding their planned surgery. It has long been the tradition to instruct patients that their surgery could be canceled if they fail to strictly follow the "nothing by mouth" (NPO) instructions. The rationale for traditional NPO guidelines was based on the risk of aspiration during anesthesia if the stomach was not empty.[14] It has long been assumed that by limiting oral intake, the stomach would be empty on the morning of surgery, thereby reducing the risk of pulmonary aspiration.

In the mid-to-late 1990s, several small studies began to surface in the literature questioning the validity of the NPO guidelines common in perioperative areas. The results of several small pragmatic studies showed that there was no difference in outcomes when patients were allowed to eat or drink up to only a few hours before their scheduled surgery. Although these results seemed promising, the studies were all underpowered to enable a global practice change.

The lack of a large, adequately powered study was the impetus behind the 2003 systematic review and meta-analysis that helped fuel practice change regarding NPO status in the perioperative period.[15] Brady and colleagues[15] showed that the risk of perioperative aspiration was no greater when less stringent NPO guidelines were used. As a result of this systematic review, many perioperative professional practice organizations revised their NPO practice guidelines.

Since the revisions to the NPO guidelines have been made, patient outcomes have remained excellent while patient satisfaction has increased. Additionally, improvements in operating room schedules, operating room throughput, rates of surgical cancellations, and patient compliance have all improved since the evidence-informed NPO guidelines were introduced into practice.[14]

SUMMARY

Perioperative care is comprised of three care components: (1) preoperative, (2) intraoperative, and (3) postoperative care. All three components are distinct, yet overlapping, and the perioperative patient moves across all three care areas. Given the vulnerable status of the perioperative patient, coupled with the complex nature of these areas, EBP and clinical decision-making that is rooted in high-quality evidence is required for safe and effective patient and family care. EBP is comprised of three critical elements: (1) patient and family preferences, (2) clinical expertise, and (3) best available evidence. Systematic reviews provide the highest quality of evidence and, fortunately, systematic reviews focusing on perioperative care issues are a growing area within the evidence literature base.

REFERENCES

1. Stannard D, Krenzischek DA. Perianesthesia nursing care: a bedside guide for safe recovery. Philadelphia: Jones & Bartlett; 2012.
2. American Society of PeriAnesthesia Nurses. Standards and guidelines with interpretive statements: 2012-2014. Cherry Hill (NJ): Author; 2012.
3. Fowler PH, Craig J, Fredendall LD, et al. Perioperative workflow: barriers to efficiency, risks, and satisfaction. AORN J 2008;87(1):187–208.
4. Lin HT, Ting PC, Chang WY, et al. Predictive risk index and prognosis of postoperative reintubation after planned extubation during general anesthesia: a

single-center retrospective case-controlled study in Taiwan from 2005 to 2009. ACTA Anaesthesiol Taiwan 2013;51(1):3–9.

5. IOM (Institute of Medicine). Finding what works in health care: standards for systematic reviews. Washington, DC: National Academies Press; 2011.

6. Burford B, Lewin S, Welch V, et al. Assessing the applicability of findings in systematic reviews of complex interventions can enhance the utility of reviews for decision making. J Clin Epidemiol 2013;66(11):1251–61.

7. Westerdahl E, Tenling A. Preoperative physical therapy reduces risk of postoperative atelectasis and pneumonia in people undergoing elective cardiac surgery. Evid Based Nurs 2014;17(1):13–4.

8. Bradt J, Dileo C, Shim M. Music interventions for preoperative anxiety. Cochrane Database Syst Rev 2013;(6):CD006908.

9. Modolo NS, Modolo MP, Marton MA, et al. Intravenous versus inhalation anaesthsia for one-lung ventilation. Cochrane Database Syst Rev 2013;(7):CD006313.

10. Bassi A, Milani W, El Dib R, et al. Intravenous versus inhalation anaesthesia for one-lung ventilation. Cochrane Database Syst Rev 2008;(2):CD006313.

11. Guay J, Choi P, Suresh S, et al. Neuraxial blockade for the prevention of postoperative mortality and major morbidity: an overview of Cochrane Systematic Reviews. Cochrane Database Syst Rev 2014;(1):CD010108.

12. Riddle D, Nugent H. Intraoperative brain activity monitoring and post-anesthesia care length of stay: a systematic review. JBI Database of Systematic Reviews and Implementation Reports 2011;9(47):1971–98.

13. Harvey LA, Brosseau L, Herbert RD. Continuous passive motion following total knee arthroplasty in people with arthritis. Cochrane Database Syst Rev 2014;(2):CD004260.

14. Murphy GS, Ault ML, Wong HY, et al. The effect of a new NPO policy on operating room utilization. J Clin Anesth 2000;12(1):48–51.

15. Brady M, Kinn S, Stuart P, et al. Preoperative fasting for adults to prevent perioperative complications. Cochrane Database Syst Rev 2003;(4):CD004423.

Evidence-Based Health Care in Pediatrics

Suzanne Robertson-Malt, PhD

KEYWORDS

- Pediatric nursing care • Evidence-based health care • Systematic reviews
- Evidence implementation

KEY POINTS

- Systematic reviews are regarded as the gold standard of evidence to guide clinical decision making.
- Given the important role that systematic reviews play in influencing the evidence base of our clinical decision making, there are international standards to be followed to ensure the quality and standards in the reporting and publication of systematic reviews.
- The development and dissemination of clinical guidelines to improve the quality of pediatric care is a frequent activity internationally. Ideally, these clinical guidelines draw on the evidence generated from high-quality systematic reviews of both qualitative and quantitative research.

INTRODUCTION

The 2013, volume 48, issue 2 of *Nursing Clinics of North America* provides an overview of evidence-based nursing strategies for children of various ages and diagnoses. Each article reflects a genuine commitment on the investigator's behalf to ensuring that the evidence arising from the best available research informs their systems and processes of care. The issue's editor, Patricia Buckhart, however, encourages the journal's readership to appreciate that more is needed to advance scientifically based interventions for assisting children and their families to successfully manage their health conditions, stating that:

> Evidence based health care continues to make important contributions to the well being of children. To ensure the paediatric community can maximize the potential use of these interventions, it is important to ensure that systematic reviews are conducted and reported at the highest possible quality. Such reviews will be of benefit to a broad spectrum of interested stakeholders.[1]

Disclosure: none.
Implementation Science, Joanna Briggs Institute, School of Translational Health Science, University of Adelaide, 1/115 Grenfell Street, Adelaide, South Australia 5000, Australia
E-mail address: suzanne.robertson-malt@adelaide.edu.au

Nurs Clin N Am 49 (2014) 493–506
http://dx.doi.org/10.1016/j.cnur.2014.08.005
0029-6465/14/$ – see front matter © 2014 Elsevier Inc. All rights reserved.
nursing.theclinics.com

So why are systematic reviews so important? The rigorous methods of synthesis that underpin systematic reviews position them as gold in the health care literature. A well-designed and conducted systematic review provides the reader (typically health care professionals [HCP]) with the critical summary, as encourage by Archibald Cochrane, of all research (published and unpublished) related to the question of concern.[2] According to Joanna Briggs Institute,[3] the term *evidence* in a systematic review is used to mean "the basis of belief; the substantiation or confirmation that is needed in order to believe that something is true."[3(p45)] The evidence presented from a well-conducted systematic review can be used to develop national and/or clinical guidelines that individual organizations can then adapt in the form of clinical pathways, protocols, and policies. Although the Cochrane Collaboration has developed the science and standards associated with systematic reviews on clinical questions about effectiveness, the Joanna Briggs Institute (JBI), an associated international collaboration, has established its reputation as a leader in synthesis science for systematic reviews about the feasibility, appropriateness, and meaningfulness of the existing evidence. Increasingly appreciated among HCP is that the evidence arising from systematic reviews focused on these questions are of equal importance to questions about effectiveness as they inform HCP about the evidence base for the various social, cultural, and economic factors that impact and inform the delivery of effective and efficient health care.[3]

Given the importance of systematic reviews to the HCP, the American-based National Library of Medicine (PubMed) has designed a filter specific for the retrieval of citations indexed as systematic reviews. Using this filter, combined with the search term *pediatrics*, a total of 5340 citations were identified covering the dates from 1967 to October 2013. **Table 1** provides a summary of this search.

Of particular note when reviewing the data presented in **Table 1** is that only 18% of these publications are systematic reviews. The majority are literature reviews, guidelines, or consensus statements from professional societies, such as the American Academy of Pediatrics or the European Society for Pediatrics, and so forth. A total of 14.2% are literature reviews of a clinical question or topic. Sometimes the word *systematic* is still used to describe these literature reviews, which can be misleading to the uniformed reader. Just because a publication uses the term *systematic review* does not mean that it has followed the 7-step process (**Table 2**) of synthesis science upheld by either JBI or Cochrane. Hodson and Craig[4] emphasize this point in their 2013 publication on systematic reviews of pediatric nephrology with the following statement:

> The term "systematic review" does not guarantee that a review covers all the available data, that the validity of included studies has been appropriately assessed, or that data have been combined appropriately in meta-analyses.[4(p197)]

THE IMPORTANCE OF QUALITY IN REPORTING AND PUBLISHING SYSTEMATIC REVIEWS

Across all health care specialties, including pediatrics, the number of systematic reviews being published has increased since 1976 with almost an exponential trend. However, the clarity and transparency of these publications is not always optimal. The search methods with regard to the types of databases, additional sources, and the number of databases searched differ widely across systematic reviews. MEDLINE is often the most commonly used database and often the only database searched.

Table 1
Summary of publications: 1967 to October 2013

Type of Publication	Total Number	Total (%)	Sample Titles
Systematic reviews	987	18	• Universal mental health screening in pediatric primary care: a systematic review • Evidence for family centered care for children with special health care needs: a systematic review • A systematic review of the literature on evaluative studies of tonsillectomy and adenoidectomy
Meta-analysis	529	10	• Predictors of recurrent febrile seizures: a meta-analytic review • The effect of day-care exposure on the risk of developing type 1 diabetes: a meta-analysis of case-control studies • Cigarette smoking-associated changes in blood lipid and lipoprotein levels in the 8- to 19-year-old age group: a meta-analysis
Combined systematic review & meta-analysis	172	3.2	• Does exercise improve glycemic control in type 1 diabetes? A systematic review and meta-analysis • Breast-feeding and the risk of bronchial asthma in childhood: a systematic review with meta-analysis of prospective studies • Probiotics to prevent or treat excessive infant crying: systematic review and meta-analysis
Guideline	394	7.3	• The implementation and evaluation of an evidence-based statewide prehospital pain management protocol developed using the national prehospital evidence-based guideline model process for emergency medical services • Clinical practice guideline: tympanostomy tubes in children • Guideline for the prevention of acute nausea and vomiting caused by antineoplastic medication in pediatric patients with cancer
Consensus statements	389	7.3	• Recommendations for self-monitoring in pediatric diabetes: a consensus statement by the Italian Society of Pediatric Endocrinology and Diabetology • Quality metrics in neonatal and pediatric critical care transport: a consensus statement • Consensus statement of the Indian Academy of Pediatrics on integrated management of severe acute malnutrition
Literature review	757	14.2	• Acute pediatric facial nerve paralysis as the first indication for familial cerebral cavernoma: case presentation and literature review • Correlation between socioeconomic indicators and traumatic dental injuries: a qualitative critical literature review • Abusive head trauma in children: a literature review

Table 2	
Seven steps of conducting a systematic review	
Step	**Process**
1	The development of a rigorous proposal or protocol setting a predetermined plan to ensure scientific rigor and minimize potential bias
2	Stating the review questions hypothesis
3	Establishing the criteria that will be used to select the literature
4	Detailing a strategy to identify all relevant literature from an agreed time frame
5	Critical appraisal of the studies retrieved
6	Extracting data from the primary research regarding the participants, the intervention/issue or phenomena of interest, the outcomes, and results
7	Generating a summary (meta-analysis or meta-aggregation) or descriptive narrative of the results

Adapted from Joanna Briggs Institute Reviewers' manual: 2011 edition. Joanna Briggs Institute, The University of Adelaide. p. 45–76; with permission.

Lundh and colleagues[5] concluded the same in their 2009 systematic review of the quality of systematic reviews in pediatric oncology:

> *most systematic reviews in the field of paediatric oncology seem to have serious methodological flaws across all domains leading to a high risk of bias.*[5(p651)]

This concern over the quality of systematic reviews is by no means unique to the specialty of pediatrics. Poor reporting of systematic reviews diminishes their value to clinicians, policy makers, and other users. Given the disparity in the quality of published systematic reviews, an international group of experienced investigators and methodologists developed what is now considered the international standard: PRISMA (*P*referred *R*eporting *I*tems for *S*ystematic Reviews and *M*eta-*A*nalyses) for the report and publication of systematic reviews.[6] In seeking the best available evidence to inform the systems and processes of pediatric care, it is important to appreciate these standards. Exaggerated and biased results from poorly designed and reported studies can trigger their premature dissemination and lead HCP into making incorrect treatment decisions.[7]

Table 3 provides a high-level overview of systematic reviews in the specialty of pediatrics since 1989 addressing a broad range of question types. Of note is the fact that even with the introduction of the PRISMA standards in 2005, the quality of reporting continues to vary. Thus, readers should read a systematic review carefully before accepting its results and conclusions.

It is important to appreciate that the breakdown in the quality of evidence being reported does not start with systematic reviews. Too often, systematic reviews conclude with the statement that the existing research base is limited for use in practice because of poorly designed and reported outcomes. (**Table 4** provides an example of these concluding statements.) Dr Richard Horton, in his plenary address to the audience of the first summit of the Standards for Research in Child Health (StaR), emphasized that

> *A lack of research, poor research, and poorly reported research are violations of children's human rights.*[14(p3112)]

The StaR Child Health initiative was founded in 2009 in an effort to address a growing concern within the pediatric research community about the poor standards

Table 3
Samples of systematic reviews in specialty of pediatrics

Date	Sample Titles	Purpose of Systematic Review	Limitations of PRISMA Standards	Type of Question
1989	"Corticosteroids as Adjunctive Therapy in Bacterial Meningitis. A Meta-Analysis of Clinical Trials"[8]	The benefit of corticosteroids for adjunctive therapy for bacterial meningitis	Not details provided about inclusion/ exclusion criteria; database search strategy; critical appraisal; method of analysis	Effectiveness
1991	"The Risk of Seizure Recurrence Following a First Unprovoked Seizure: A Quantitative Review"[9]	To evaluate the strength of association	Not details provided about inclusion/ exclusion criteria; database search strategy; critical appraisal; method of analysis	Prognostic
1997	"The Use of Antibiotics to Prevent Serious Sequelae in Children at Risk for Occult Bacteremia: A Meta-analysis"[10]	To determine whether antibiotics prevent serious bacterial infections in children at risk for occult bacteremia	Limited search of available databases (1 only) No detail provided about study selection; search strategy	Effectiveness
2009	"Impact of Caring for a Child With Cerebral Palsy on the Quality of Life of Parents: A Systematic Review"[11]	To understand how research is evolving and the relevant data that should be taken into account when planning interventions with these families	Limited search of available database No detail about accessing unpublished research English-speaking-only research No standardized appraisal tool	Meaningfulness
2012	"Optimal Sedation in Pediatric Intensive Care Patients: A Systematic Review"[12]	To evaluate the reported incidences of underoptimal and oversedation in pediatric intensive care patients and to determine to what extent the goal of adequate sedation is met	Limited search of 2 databases (PubMed & EMBASE) English-language only No details about accessing gray literature/ unpublished research	Appropriateness
2013	"Medication Adherence and Health Care Utilization in Pediatric Chronic Illness: A Systematic Review"[13]	Understanding the impact of adherence promotion interventions on costs specific to pediatric populations To better understand how modifiable factors contribute to health care costs and value to identify relevant and significant priorities of health care reform	Systematic review conducted and reported in accordance with the PRISMA standards	Meaningfulness and feasibility

| Table 4 |
| Examples of evidence-based recommendations |

Patient Care Interventions	Evidence-Based Recommendations
Pharmacologic treatments	We suggest that pharmacotherapy be offered only by clinicians who are experienced in the use of antiobesity agents and are aware of the potential for adverse reactions.[9(p4586)]
Lifestyle: dietary interventions only	Eating timely, regular meals, particularly breakfast, and avoiding constant "grazing" during the day, especially after school.[9(p4584)]
Lifestyle: physical activity interventions only	We recommend that clinicians prescribe and support 60 min of daily moderate to vigorous physical activity.[9(p4592)]
Combination lifestyle interventions (physical activity and dietary modification)	We suggest that clinicians promote and participate in efforts to educate the community about healthy dietary and activity habits.[9(p4592)]

in both the design and reporting of pediatric clinical trials that, in turn, impact the quality of evidence available to guide clinical decision making. The mission of the StaR Child Health is

> To improve the design, conduct, and reporting of paediatric research through the development and dissemination of evidence-based standards. This involves a systematic "knowledge to action" process, which includes the following: identifying problems that need to be addressed; identifying and reviewing knowledge relevant to the problem; generating knowledge where gaps exist; adapting knowledge to the relevant context; assessing barriers to knowledge implementation; designing knowledge transfer strategies and promoting best practice; and evaluating knowledge uptake and the impact on practice.[14(p3112)]

The StaR Child Health global initiative is sponsored by leading pediatric health care facilities from across the globe, such as the Children's Hospital, Westmead, Australia; The Children's Hospital of Eastern Ontario Research Institute, France; and SickKids Research Institute, Canada. The first activity of the StaR Child Health initiative was to conduct a systematic search of the available research and guidance for pediatric clinical trials.[9] A modified version of the *Appraisal of Guidelines Research and Evaluation* (AGREE) instrument was used to determine the quality of the 60 documents found on the Internet: 3779 articles found in bibliographic databases, 22 Internet guideline documents, and 18 scientific publications. The appraisal of these guidelines showed that the methods undertaken to develop the existing guidelines was poor and that the quality of existing research resulted in the guidelines being limited to statements about "what one should aim to do" instead of "how to do it."[14(p3113)]

The standards being established by each of these international organizations, the StaR Child Health, PRISMA, and AGREE, point to the critical dependence that each phase of the process for evidence-based health care has on the quality conduct of the proceeding phase:

- Identifying and researching questions of urgency to patient care
- The design and reporting of research findings
- The synthesis of all research findings: systematic reviews and meta-analysis
- The development of clinical guidelines
- The implementation of evidence into everyday systems and processes of care

When clinical research is not firmly grounded in historic and contemporary patient care data, then the relevance of the research findings to the everyday treatment and management of patients is limited. Too often clinical research is designed and conducted without a careful analysis of existing research in the area and the outcomes being used to measure the feasibility, appropriateness, meaningfulness, and effectiveness of the particular intervention or strategy.

CASE STUDY

In attempting to highlight the challenge that readers face when determining the quality of published systematic reviews, the following case study will reflect on published systematic reviews in an area of pediatric health care (pediatric obesity) that is generating a lot of research and the subsequent development of systematic reviews and clinical guidelines. These reviews reflect a range of foci and criteria for inclusion that has resulted in a variety of reported outcomes, many of which are not comparable.

Halting the rising prevalence of obesity in children is considered to be a public health priority throughout the developed nations of the world. Researchers across the globe are actively studying a spectrum of strategies focused on finding answers to a whole host of questions confronting clinicians about the prevention, diagnosis, and management of childhood obesity, such as the following: Is there a particular drug effective in reducing weight gain? When should surgery be introduced in the program of management for a child's obesity? What factors influence a child's food preferences? What support strategies do families need in helping to manage a child diagnosed as obese? The publication of 8 systematic reviews (**Table 5**) over the past decade signals the urgency associated with this area of pediatric health care and the desire to determine the efficacy of more than 600 research studies and the range of strategies being proposed to manage childhood obesity.[1-7] Despite the comprehensive nature of a well-designed systematic review, no review can address all the questions of importance related to the management of pediatric obesity. Typically, the synthesis of all systematic reviews related to a health care issue/topic occurs at the time of developing a clinical guideline. However, a new generation of systematic reviews is being developed called *umbrella reviews* or *overview of reviews*. The science base for this new type

Table 5
Systematic reviews: pediatric obesity

Date	Title
2013	"Impact of Physical Activity Intervention Programs on Self-efficacy in Youths: A Systematic Review"[15]
2010	"Efficacy and Safety of Anti-obesity Drugs in Children and Adolescents: Systematic Review and Meta-analysis"[16]
2008	"Behavioral Interventions to Prevent Childhood Obesity: A Systematic Review and Meta-analyses of Randomized Trial"[17]
2008	"Treatment of Pediatric Obesity: A Systematic Review and Meta-analysis of Randomized Trials"[18]
2006	"Efficacy of Exercise for Treating Overweight in Children and Adolescents: A Systematic Review"[19]
2005	"Pharmacologic Treatment of Obesity"[20]
2003	"Long-term Pharmacotherapy for Overweight and Obesity: A Systematic Review and Meta-analysis of Randomized Controlled Trials"[21]
2001	"Meta-analysis: Pharmacologic Treatment of Obesity"[22]

of review is still in its infancy. Despite there being 8 systematic reviews for pediatric obesity, an umbrella review does not, as yet, exist.

In 2008, McGovern and colleagues[18] completed a systematic review for the Endocrine Society Pediatric Obesity Task Force. The results of the systematic review, in turn, informed the development of the society's clinical practice guideline published in 2008:

> The Endocrine Society decided to formulate clinical practice guidelines for the management of paediatric obesity. In doing so, it formed a Task Force to develop these recommendations. This Task Force asked the Mayo Knowledge and Encounter Research Unit, under contract to perform evidence syntheses with The Endocrine Society, to conduct a systematic review of the literature on the treatment of paediatric obesity. This report briefly summarizes the findings of a systematic review and meta-analyses of randomized trials published in the literature up to February 2006 and reports on the effect of evaluated treatments on obesity outcomes.[18(p4601)]

In the 2008 the publication of their systematic review, McGovern and colleagues[18] indicate that they

> produced this report in adherence with the Quality of Reporting of Meta-analyses (QUOROM) standards for reporting systematic reviews of randomized trials.[18(p4601)]

The QUOROM standards are the first iteration of the PRISMA standards. The 7 steps for conducting a systematic review referred to in **Table 2** closely align with the PRISMA standards and are used to present McGovern and colleagues'[18] systematic review and the process they followed.

Step 1: The Development of a Rigorous Proposal or Protocol Setting a Predetermined Plan to Ensure Scientific Rigor and Minimize Potential Bias

The protocol becomes a map that guides the review author's systematic search of the existing research. McGovern and colleagues[18] commence their systematic review under the guidance of an expert peer review group composed of both clinical and research/methodology experts in pediatric obesity:

> The Endocrine Society Paediatric Obesity Task Force commissioned this review, approved the review protocol, offered references, and provided insight into the interpretation of the results.[18(p4601)]

This peer review proves an invaluable means of ensuring that there are no omissions that could result in introducing bias into the review process and subsequent reporting of results.

Step 2: Stating the Review Questions Hypothesis

McGovern and colleauges'[9] protocol includes a clearly defined question that aligns with the PICO (Population, Intervention, Comparison, Outcome) acronym upheld by both JBI and Cochrane:

- Population: overweight children and adolescents
- Intervention: nonsurgical interventions (diet, physical activity, and pharmacologic agents)
- Comparison: no details provided
- Outcome: weight loss

Step 3: Establishing the Criteria That Will Be Used to Select the Literature

The protocol also includes details about the inclusion and exclusion criteria. This information is essential in helping the reader to familiarize with the scope and limitations of the review. The inclusion criteria not only refer to the participants (age, comorbidities, and so forth) but also the study design:

> *Eligible studies were fully published randomized trials (in any language) with the majority of participants being overweight (as defined in each study) children and adolescents (ages 2–18) and assessing the effect of lifestyle and pharmacological interventions on obesity outcomes.*[18(p4602)]

The eligible interventions

> *Eligible lifestyle interventions included any treatment strategy aimed at changing the diet and/or activity level of overweight children…*

> *Eligible pharmacological interventions were medications used with the objective of reducing obesity measures in overweight children.*[18(p4602)]

The exclusion criteria

> *we excluded trials of patients with type 1 diabetes or eating disorders (bulimia or anorexia nervosa), Prader-Willi patients, and other patients in which obesity is part of a clinical syndrome and follows different natural and clinical histories.*[18(p4602)]

The outcome measurements of interest

> *Eligible studies assessed an objective mass-based obesity measurement at the end of the study period (regardless of whether authors reported the results of the intervention on this measure).*[18(p4602)]

Step 4: Detailing a Strategy to Identify All Relevant Literature from an Agreed Time Frame

McGovern and colleagues[18] provide the reader with comprehensive details about what databases were searched and the search strategy used. Such information helps the reader to develop an appreciation for how exhaustive the search was for all available research on the question at hand. Bias is easily introduced into the systematic review at this stage by limiting the search to 1 or 2 databases and/or only journals that publish in English language. According to the standards upheld by the Cochrane Collaboration

> *review authors are recommended to search trial registers, conference abstracts, grey literature, etc, as well as standard bibliographic databases such as MEDLINE, PUBMED, EMBASE. It is argued that a systematic review needs to search comprehensively in order to avoid publication biases (section 13.3.1.1).*[23]

The fact that review authors limit the number of databases searched but still follow a rigorous protocol has resulted in a subtle shift in classification occurring within the literature with the term *comprehensive* being added to the review title if their search strategy included a wide range of subject matter databases. Despite this classification occurring within the published literature, consensus on this change among the leading organizations, such as JBI, Cochrane, and Campbell, has not been achieved.

Review authors are encouraged to seek direction in the design of their search strategy from a Medical librarian. McGovern and colleagues[18] commence their discussion on the identification and retrieval of all research that meets their inclusion and exclusion criteria by referring to the assistance they obtained for the development of their search strategy from both an expert librarian and from and a team of pediatric physicians and researchers:

> *An expert reference librarian (P.J.E.) designed and conducted the electronic search strategy with input from a team of paediatric physicians and researchers. To identify eligible studies, our systematic search included the electronic databases MEDLINE, EMBASE, ERIC, CINAHL, Cochrane Central Register of Controlled Trials (CENTRAL), PSYCInfo, Dissertation Abstracts International, Science Citation Index, and Social Science Citation Index, in all cases from their inception until February 2006 (detailed search strategies available from the authors). We also reviewed the reference sections of identified reviews and published guidelines. Finally, we received suggestions for inclusion of articles from paediatric obesity experts that comprised The Endocrine Society Paediatric Obesity Task Force.[18(p4601)]*

A total of 1162 abstracts were identified from their initial search, and 889 were excluded following a review of both the title and abstract. The full texts of the remaining 263 studies were accessed for more careful review. McGovern and colleagues[18] minimized bias in the selection of potential studies for inclusion by having more than 1 member of the review team complete this process independently. When a difference of opinion arose, which could not be resolved through discussion, a third person was called on to make a resolution:

> *One team of two reviewers (L.M. and C.C.K.) independently identified for full text retrieval all eligible records from the abstracts and titles; records in which the reviewers disagreed were also retrieved in full text. Teams of two reviewers (L.M., R.P., and A.H.) working independently and in duplicate again reviewed the full text articles for eligibility; an endocrinologist with expertise in research methodology (V.M.M.) not involved in the initial assessment resolved disagreements.[18(p4602)]*

This process of search and selection of potential studies for inclusion is presented as a graphic (the PRISMA flow diagram) in McGovern and colleagues'[18] publication, which is a key requirement of the PRISMA standards.

Step 5: Critical Appraisal of the Studies Retrieved

McGovern and colleagues[18] used a standardized critical appraisal tool to facilitate the determination of the methodological quality of the included studies. Given that McGovern and colleagues'[18] systematic review is about effectiveness and, therefore, only included randomized controlled trials (RCTs), the appraisal they followed focused on the criteria critical to determining the internal and external validity of each included RCT:

> *To ascertain the validity of eligible randomized trials, pairs of reviewers working independently and with substantial reliability (corresponding k where appropriate) determined the extent to which trials reported concealment of allocation (k=0.94), blinding of patients (k=0.94) to the provider of intervention (k=0.94) and data collectors (k=1), blinding to the hypothesis (k=1), level of randomization (k=0.83), and extent of loss to follow-up (i.e. the percentage of patients in whom the investigators were not able to ascertain outcomes).[18(p4601)]*

Presenting the results of the critical appraisal provides the reader with an opportunity to determine the overall methodological quality of the included studies.

Unfortunately, as discussed in the beginning sections of this article, the conduct and reporting of clinical research is not always optimal, resulting in the article receiving a low ranking for methodological quality as occurred in McGovern and colleagues'[18] review:

> *Almost all trials across these reviews lacked reporting or conduct of allocation concealment and blinding (except for placebo-controlled drug trials); nearly half of the trials lost 10% or more participants to follow-up (i.e. had no outcome data at the end of trial for these randomized participants).*[18(p4602)]

Critical appraisal is central to moving the interpretation of the results of a study from statistical significance to clinical significance. Often a study can be statistically significant but not clinically significant. To arrive at a position regarding clinical significance, the review authors must determine the generalizability (the external validity) of individual study results. Pearson and colleagues[24] suggest that when determining clinical significance, the review authors need to ask the following:

> *...Is the population I am interested in so different from those in the study that the results don't apply? You need to consider whether or not the results can be generalized to a wider population and/or to your own patients specifically.*[24(p10)]

Step 6: Extracting Data from the Primary Research Regarding the Participants, the Intervention/Issue or Phenomena of Interest, the Outcomes, and Results

To minimize error in the data extracted from the included studies, McGovern and colleagues[18] maintained their process of independent, duplicate review using a data extraction sheet to guide and reinforce the type of data needed:

> *Working in duplicate, six trained reviewers extracted the following data from each eligible article: year and journal of publication, type of study (e.g. pilot), level of randomization (e.g. community, school, or clinical), participants (age and gender), measure of obesity (BMI, percent overweight, percent fat-free mass, or visceral adiposity), experimental and control interventions (type of intervention, deliverer of intervention, and level and duration of intervention) and results....*[18(p4601)]

Step 7: Generating a Summary (Meta-analysis or Meta-aggregation) or Descriptive Narrative of the Results

From the systematic process of searching the subject matter databases and determining if the study met the inclusion and exclusion criteria outlined in the initial protocol, a total of 76 studies were included in the systematic review, with 61 of these included in a variety of meta-analyses. Each of the primary outcomes of interest identified in McGovern and colleagues'[18] protocol are reported on

1. Pharmacologic interventions
   a. Seventeen studies met the inclusion/exclusion criteria.
   b. Nine studies were included in a meta-analysis.
2. Dietary interventions
   a. Six studies met the inclusion/exclusion criteria.
   b. Six studies were included in a meta-analysis.
3. Physical activity interventions
   a. Twenty studies met the inclusion/exclusion criteria.
   b. Seventeen studies were included in a meta-analysis.
4. Combined lifestyle interventions

a. Thirty studies met the inclusion/exclusion criteria.
b. Twenty-three studies were included in a meta-analysis.

This differentiation between studies meeting inclusion/exclusion criteria for the systematic review versus studies included in a meta-analysis is a concept that can often become confusing to the reader. It is not uncommon for a clinician to think that systematic reviews and meta-analysis are one and the same thing, that is, have the same definition. This belief is a categorical error. Meta-analysis is a statistical method for the pooling of data. This pooling of data, however, should only occur if the combined studies are similar (homogenous) (ie, clinical, methodological, and/or statistical). There are a variety of methods to assess primary study heterogeneity commencing with a graphic display of the included studies called a forest plot. This is followed by a statistical analysis that both JBI and Cochrane recommend: the I^2 index. The I^2 statistical is reported as a percentage with the following guidance provided by Higgins and Green[23] for interpreting I^2:

- 0% = no heterogeneity
- 25% = low heterogeneity
- 50% = moderate heterogeneity
- 75% = high heterogeneity

The level of heterogeneity in McGovern and colleagues'[18(p4603)] meta-analysis ranged from 0% to 30% for trials within the pharmacy interventions outcome, 22.5% in the dietary interventions only, and 29% in the physical activity interventions only. The results from McGovern and colleagues'[18] systematic review and meta-analysis, along with other systematic reviews on the subject, helped to inform The Endocrine Society's formulation of 65 evidence-based recommendations for the prevention, assessment, and management of pediatric obesity (see **Table 4** for examples).

SUMMARY

The development and dissemination of clinical guidelines to improve the quality of pediatric care is a frequent activity internationally. Ideally, these clinical guidelines draw on the evidence generated from high-quality systematic reviews of both qualitative and quantitative research. However, this article attempts to highlight to the reader the importance of being cautious in their consumption of the evidence-based literature. The reader needs to develop a healthy skepticism that understands that just because a publication uses *systematic review* or *clinical guideline* in the title does not ensure it is reporting quality results. Increasingly, peer-reviewed journals are adopting the international standards for the reporting and/or publication of clinical research (different standards according to the method), systematic reviews, and clinical guidelines. However, until such time as this becomes common practice, it is important for the reader to be familiar with these minimum expectations to ensure they use the best available evidence in their everyday care of pediatric patients.

REFERENCES

1. Burkhart P. Current challenges in paediatric. Nurs Clin North Am 2013;48(2): xiii–xiv.
2. Cochrane AL. Foreword. In: Chalmers I, Enkin M, Keirse MJ, editors. Effective care in pregnancy and childbirth. Oxford (England): Oxford University Press; 1989. p. i–ii.

3. Joanna Briggs Institute Reviewers' manual: 2011 edition. Joanna Briggs Institute, The University of Adelaide.
4. Hodson E, Craig J. The contribution of systematic reviews to the practice of paediatric nephrology. Pediatr Nephrol 2013;28:197–206.
5. Lundh A, Knijnenburg S, Jorgensen A, et al. Quality of systematic reviews in paediatric oncology- a systematic review. Cancer Treat Rev 2009;35:645–52.
6. Liberati A, Altman D, Tetzlaff J, et al. Research methods & reporting: the PRISMA statement for reporting systematic reviews and meta-analyses of studies that evaluate healthcare interventions: explanation and elaboration. BMJ 2009;339: b2700.
7. Moher D, Tetziaff J, Tricco A, et al. Epidemiology and reporting characteristics of systematic reviews. PLoS Med 2007;4(3):e78.
8. Havens P, Wendelberger L, Hoffman G, et al. Corticosteroids as adjunctive therapy in bacterial meningitis. A meta-analysis of clinical trials. Am J Dis Child 1989; 143(9):1051–5.
9. Berger A, Shinnar S. The risk of seizure recurrence following a first unprovoked seizure: a quantitative review. Neurology 1991;41(7):965–72.
10. Bulloch B, Craig W, Klassen T. The use of antibiotics to prevent serious sequelae in children at risk for occult bacteremia: a meta-analysis. Acad Emerg Med 1997; 4(7):679–83.
11. Pousada M, Guillamon N, Hernandez-Encuenetra E, et al. Impact of caring for a child with cerebral palsy on the quality of life of parents: a systematic review of the literature. J Dev Phys Disabil 2013;25(5):545–77.
12. Vet NJ, Ista E, de Wildt S, et al. Optimal sedation in pediatric intensive care patients: a systematic review. Intensive Care Med 2013;39(9):1524–34.
13. McGrady M, Hommel K. Medication adherence and health care utilization in pediatric chronic illness: a systematic review. Pediatrics 2013;132(4):730–40.
14. Frakking F, van der Lee J, Klassen T, et al. Report: survey of current guidance for child health clinical trials. 2009. Available at: www.starchildhealth.org. Accessed October 22, 2014.
15. Cataldo R, John J, Chandran L, et al. Impact of physical activity intervention programs on self-efficacy in youths: a systematic review. ISRN Obes 2013;2013: 586497.
16. Viner R, Hsia Y, Tmsic T, et al. Efficacy and safety of anti-obesity drugs in children and adolescents: systematic review and meta-analysis. Obes Rev 2010;11: 593–602.
17. Kamath C, Vickers K, Ehrlich A, et al. Behavioral interventions to prevent childhood obesity: a systematic review and meta-analyses of randomized trials. J Clin Endocrinol Metab 2008;93:4606–15.
18. McGovern L, Johnson J, Paulo R, et al. Treatment of pediatric obesity: a systematic review and meta-analysis of randomized trials. J Clin Endocrinol Metab 2008; 93:4600–5.
19. Atlantis E, Barnes E, Singh F. Efficacy of exercise for treating overweight in children and adolescents: a systematic review. Int J Obes 2006;30:1027–40.
20. Padwal R, Li S, Lau D. Long-term pharmacotherapy for overweight and obesity: a systematic review and meta-analysis of randomized controlled trials. Int J Obes Relat Metab Disord 2003;27(12):1437–46.
21. Li Z, Maglione M, Tu W, et al. Meta-analysis: pharmacologic treatment of obesity. Ann Intern Med 2005;142:532–46.
22. Campbell K, Waters E, O'Meara S, et al. Interventions for preventing obesity in childhood. A systematic review. Obes Rev 2001;2:149–57.

23. [updated March 2011]. In: Higgins JP, Green S, editors. Cochrane handbook for systematic reviews of interventions version 5.1.0. The Cochrane Collaboration; 2011. Available at: www.cochrane-handbook.org.
24. Pearson A, Loveday H, Holopainen A. Critically appraising evidence for healthcare. Philadelphia: Lippincott Williams & Wilkins; 2012.

Finding and Using Best Evidence for Rehabilitation

 CrossMark

Susan W. Salmond, EdD, RN[a],*, Cheryl Holly, EdD, RN[b],
Jane Smith, DNP, RN[c]

KEYWORDS

- Systematic review • Evidence-based health care • Rehabilitation • Delirium
- Hip fracture

KEY POINTS

- Systematic reviews use different approaches to synthesize or pool data from critically appraised published and unpublished studies on a focused clinical question, ultimately providing a comprehensive summary of evidence that should be used in clinical decision making.
- A structured approach to searching for systematic reviews should be used for efficiency and efficacy.
- Evidence summaries from systematic reviews can provide critical data for identifying risk factors, screening, and prevention of delirium in postoperative hip fracture patients.

Evidence-based practice is a decision-making approach in which clinicians integrate best research evidence with their clinical expertise, the patient's preferences and values, and the clinical context to achieve the best patient outcomes.[1] With the demand for improved experiences of care, improved outcomes, and greater efficiency/lower costs, the need for an evidence-based approach to care in rehabilitation settings has never been more urgent. However, with 1500 new scientific articles added to MEDLINE each day and more than a 460% increase in the past 30 years (3376 to 18,928) in the annual number of publications using the term "rehabilitation" alone,[2] it is impossible for even the most skilled rehabilitation nurse to keep current with research; hence the need for systematic reviews. A high-quality systematic review summarizes the best

The authors have nothing to disclose.
[a] Northeast Institute for Evidence Translation and Synthesis, Rutgers School of Nursing, 65 Bergen Street, Suite 1141, Newark, NJ 07107, USA; [b] Northeast Institute for Evidence Translation and Synthesis, Rutgers School of Nursing, 65 Bergen Street, Suite 1136, Newark, NJ 07107, USA; [c] Morristown Memorial Hospital, Ortho/Trauma, 100 Madison Avenue, Morristown, NJ 07962, USA
* Corresponding author.
E-mail address: salmonsu@sn.rutgers.edu

available research on a specific topic, which results in a key source of information for healthcare system decision-making and determining clinical healthcare policy, and should include a set of recommendations to optimize patient care.[3,4] This article discusses how to find the best available evidence for rehabilitation settings and then demonstrates the use of best available evidence through a high-impact case study: delirium in an elderly patient with hip fracture.

Systematic reviews, a secondary form of research, use different approaches to synthesize or pool data from critically appraised published and unpublished studies on a focused clinical question, ultimately providing a comprehensive summary of evidence. From this summary, recommendations for care, or best practice, emerge. For example, a nurse working with adult clients with low back pain may be asked whether there would be any value to participating in a yoga class. A review of individual studies would find different sample sizes with often conflicting results, some saying it works, some saying it does not. The clinician is left confused. However, a well-designed systematic review can retrieve a comprehensive scope of publications from multiple data bases, as well as unpublished studies. These studies are critically appraised for scientific rigor, so that the final review includes studies that both match the query's criteria and are deemed scientifically reliable. Using a systematic review eliminates the need to read each individual study and attempt to draw conclusions. In this case, a search of the Cochrane database is an appropriate starting point because yoga is considered an intervention, and the Cochrane Library focuses predominantly on systematic reviews of therapy or therapeutic intervention. This search found a study protocol entitled yoga treatment of chronic nonspecific low back pain' that had been published, although the full review was not yet complete.[5] A search of MEDLINE, the database of the National Library of Medicine, using the keywords "yoga," "low-back pain," and "systematic review" found 2 systematic reviews addressing the topic. Both reviews were critically appraised using the Critical Appraisal Skills Programme tool for appraising systematic reviews (http://www.casp-uk.nt/). The article entitled "A Systematic Review and Meta-analysis of Yoga for Low Back Pain" by Cramer and colleagues[6] met the criteria for rigor using this tool. These investigators reported the impact of yoga exercise on key patient-centered outcomes and found strong evidence for short-term effects on pain, back-specific disability, and global improvement. There was also strong evidence for a long-term effect on pain, and moderate evidence for a long-term effect on back-specific disability. Based on this evidence, the nurse in our example would recommend yoga exercise to this client and should consider developing resources on available classes to promote to other clients.

WHERE TO FIND SYSTEMATIC REVIEWS

A methodical search moving from synopses to databases is likely to be the most efficient and efficacious approach for finding the evidence and is summarized in **Table 1**.[7]

Synopses

For busy clinicians, a beginning point may be to search for synopses of systematic reviews. Synopses of systematic reviews are short summaries providing a critical appraisal of the science along with a brief examination of the evidence. Synopses are published in journals such as *Evidence Based Nursing*, *International Journal of Evidence-Based Healthcare*, and *ACP Journal Club*. A Web site providing synopses of systematic reviews is the Database of Abstracts of Reviews of Effectiveness (DARE). The DARE site focuses solely on studies of effectiveness. Using DARE to research back pain, a total of 334 synopses were identified focusing on a range of interventions such as back schools, herbal medicine, behavioral treatment, prolotherapy injections, chiropractic interventions, and massage.

Organizations Producing Systematic Reviews

In the absence of synopses, the next search should be independent organizations that produce systematic reviews. These organizations include the Cochrane Library, Campbell Collaboration, and Joanna Briggs Institute for Nursing and Midwifery (JBI). Each of these organizations has a different focus. The Cochrane Library predominantly provides systematic reviews targeting therapy or effectiveness research. Different Cochrane review groups of interest to rehabilitation practitioners are likely to be the back group; bone, joint, and muscle trauma group; dementia and cognitive improvement group; injuries group; musculoskeletal group; neuromuscular disease group; pain, palliative, and supportive care group; and the stroke group. Effectiveness reviews limit the study methodology to randomized controlled trials (RCTs) and case-control trials because they represent the gold standard for studies of effectiveness. However, in many areas of nursing and rehabilitation there is a dearth of studies examining effectiveness using RCTs.

JBI is an international research network providing evidence-based resources including systematic reviews and evidence summaries. JBI has developed systematic review methodologies for synthesizing multiple types of study designs. These reviews may be of quantitative or qualitative research data, text, and/or opinion, and may relate to economic data or combinations of these. By not limiting the research method approach to RCTs, it is possible to address research questions beyond that of effectiveness. Moreover, for questions of effectiveness for which there are no RCTs, using alternative approaches that take the best available evidence limits the likelihood of arriving at an empty review. Schlosser and Sigafos[8] describe an empty review as one in which there are virtually no conclusions and no clinical recommendations, but rather a statement that there is insufficient evidence to answer the question.

The JBI approach is more inclusive in study design, and best available evidence captures all forms of rigorous research and experience. To this end JBI has developed multiple approaches for quantitative systematic reviews (including RCTs and other quantitative designs) and qualitative systematic reviews. Titles such as "A Systematic Review of Differences Between Brain Temperature and Core Body Temperature in Adult Patients with Severe Traumatic Brain Injury," "Interventions for Improving Coordination of Axial Segments and Lower Limbs During Walking Following Stroke: Systematic Review," and "The Psychosocial Spiritual Experience of Elderly Individuals Recovering From Stroke: A Systematic Review" are just a few of the titles drawn from the JBI library that may be of interest to the rehabilitation clinician.

The Campbell Collaboration (known as C2), another international research network producing systematic reviews, focuses on review of social intervention and services covering areas of social justice, education, and social welfare. The Campbell Library is a good place to search for systematic review on disparities, sexual abuse, drug abuse, vocational rehabilitation, and return-to-work programs. The National Center for the Dissemination of Disability Research (NCDDR) has established a partnership with "key representatives from the Campbell Collaboration to establish a Disability Research Coordinating Group that provides an infrastructure for conducting and disseminating systematic reviews" (http://www.ncddr.org/about.html).

Systematic Review Registries

Registries provide an easy way to search for systematic reviews. One registry of significant interest to those working in the area of rehabilitation is the Registry of

Table 1
Searching for systematic reviews

Synopses	
DARE	Database of abstracts of reviews providing synopses of systematic reviews that evaluate the effects of heath care interventions and the delivery and organization of health services http://www.crd.york.ac.uk/CRDWeb/
Organizations Producing Systematic Reviews	
Campbell Collaboration	An international research network focusing on developing systematic reviews targeting social interventions on policies and services in the areas of education, social welfare, and crime and justice http://www.campbellcollaboration.org/library.php
Cochrane Library	An international research network focusing on producing systematic reviews targeting therapeutic interventions. The library has more than 5000 published protocols and completed reviews www.cochrane.org
Joanna Briggs Institute (JBI)	An international research network within the School of Translational Science at the University of Adelaide, South Australia. The JBI library provides protocols, completed systematic reviews, best practice articles, and evidence summaries capturing all forms of quantitative and qualitative research www.joannabriggs.edu.au
EPPI Center	The EPPI Centre conducts systematic reviews across a range of different topic areas and provides support for others who are undertaking systematic reviews or using research evidence in the areas of health promotion, public health, and social welfare https://eppi.ioe.ac.uk/cms/
Systematic Review Registries	
Registry of Systematic Reviews of Disability and Rehabilitation Research	A central repository for systematic reviews of research studies on disability and rehabilitation topics relevant to researchers, persons with disabilities, their families, and service providers. Provided by The National Center for the Dissemination of Disability Research http://www.ktdrr.org/systematicregistry/about.html
Systematic Review Data Repository	Available through the AHRQ, this registry is an open and searchable archive of systematic reviews and their data as well as a tool for building systematic reviews http://srdr.ahrq.gov/

Prospero	Sponsored by the University of York and the National Institutes of Health Research, this comprehensive registry of protocols and completed reviews is an easily searchable source of evidence-based data http://www.crd.york.ac.uk/PROSPERO/
Databases	
CINAHL	About 3000 nursing and allied health journals are represented in this database. Allows for an advanced search in which systematic reviews can be specified under publication type
MEDLINE	MEDLINE is the US National Library of Medicine's premier bibliographic database that contains more than 19 million references to journal articles in life sciences http://www.ncbi.nlm.nih.gov/pubmed
PubMed	PubMed comprises more than 23 million citations for biomedical literature from MEDLINE, life science journals, and online books. Use the Clinical Queries function to enter "systematic reviews"
PEDro Physiotherapy Evidence Database	A database for physiotherapy with more than 26,000 randomized trials, systematic reviews, and clinical practice guidelines. All trials on PEDro are independently assessed for quality. Typing "systematic reviews" in the search box produces a list of all systematic reviews, or type the topic and "systematic review" http://www.pedro.org.au/
PsycBITE	PsycBITE is a database capturing studies of cognitive, behavioral, and other treatments for psychological problems and issues occurring as a consequence of ABI. Trials have been independently assessed for quality. Typing "systematic reviews" in the search box produces a list of all systematic reviews or type the topic and "systematic review"
PsycINFO	A database from the American Psychological Association capturing peer-reviewed articles in psychology and related disciplines. Typing "systematic reviews" in the search box produces a list of all systematic reviews or type the topic and "systematic review" www.apa.org/psycinfo
OT Seeker	Contains abstracts of systematic reviews, randomized controlled trials, and other resources relevant to OT interventions. Most trials have been critically appraised for their validity and interpretability. Typing "systematic reviews" in the search box produces a list of all systematic reviews or type the topic and "systematic review" http://www.otseeker.com/
OTDBASE	OT indexing and search service that contains more than 10,000 abstracts from more than 20 global OT journals since 1970 www.otdbase.org
OT Search	OT Search is a subscription service to a bibliographic database through the American Occupational Therapy Association. It covers the literature of OT and its related subject areas http://www1.aota.org/otsearch/

(continued on next page)

Table 1
(continued)

SpeechBITE	Speech pathology database for best interventions and treatment efficacy. Type "systematic review" in the search, or a key word and "systematic review" http://speechbite.com/
Professional/Trade Associations	
American Speech-Language-Hearing Association	Web site provides an annual list of systematic reviews, appraised for quality and relevant to speech, language, and hearing issues http://www.asha.org/members/reviews.aspx
ABIEBR	The ABIEBR is a project to develop an evidence-based review of the literature for rehabilitation or rehabilitation-related interventions for ABI. The principle of the ABIEBR is to improve the quality of ABI rehabilitation by synthesizing the current literature into a usable format and laying the foundation for effective knowledge transfer to improve programs and services http://www.abiebr.com/
NIDRR	The NIDRR Program Database includes more than 2500 current and completed projects funded by the National Institute on Disability and Rehabilitation Research from 1986 to the present. It is searchable using the term "systematic review"
Social Care Institute for Excellence	Organization dedicated to improving the lives of people who use care services through sharing knowledge. Many of these social care services are of interest to people with disabilities. Type "systematic review" into the search box
SCIRE Project	SCIRE is a synthesis of the research evidence underlying rehabilitation interventions to improve the health of people living with spinal cord injury http://www.scireproject.com/
CIRRIE	CIRRIE's mission is to share information and expertise in rehabilitation research. The CIRRIE Database of International Rehabilitation Research currently contains more than 145,000 citations of international rehabilitation research published between 1990 and the present. Type in a key word and "systematic review"

Guidelines	
American Academy Orthopedic Surgeons	Multiple clinical guidelines for common orthopedic conditions http://www.aaos.org/Research/guidelines/guide.asp
G-I-N	Organization dedicated to strengthening and supporting collaboration in guideline development, adaptation and implementation http://www.g-i-n.net/
National Guidelines Clearinghouse	Access to clinical guidelines along with ability to evaluate the guidelines www.guideline.gov
Scottish Intercollegiate Network	Access to evidence-based clinical guidelines developed by multidisciplinary working groups http://www.sign.ac.uk/
ADAPTE	Working groups from G-I-N that use a systematic approach to the endorsement and/or modification of guidelines produced in one cultural and organizational setting for application in a different context. Adaptation may be used as an alternative to de novo guideline development; eg, for customizing existing guidelines to suit the local context http://www.g-i-n.net/working-groups/adaptation
Consortium for Spinal Cord Medicine	Supported by Paralyzed Veterans of America and other professional and consumer groups, the mission centers around the development of evidence-based clinical practice guidelines that expert methodologists have graded for their scientific strength and validity http://www.pva.org/site/c.ajIRK9NJLcJ2E/b.6431479/k.3D9E/Consortium_for_Spinal_Cord_Medicine.htm

Abbreviations: ABI, acquired brain impairment; ABIEBR, Evidence-based Review of Moderate To Severe Acquired Brain Injury; AHRQ, Agency for Healthcare Research and Quality; CINAHL, Cumulative Index to Nursing and Allied Health Literature; CIRRIE, Center for International Rehabilitation Research Information and Exchange; DARE, Database of Abstracts of Reviews of Effectiveness; EPPI, Evidence for Policy and Practice Information and Coordinating; G-I-N, Guidelines International Network; JBI, Joanna Briggs Institute for Nursing and Midwifery; NIDRR, National Rehabilitation Information Center; OT, occupational therapy; Prospero, Prospective Register of Systematic Reviews; SCIRE, Spinal Cord Injury Rehabilitation Evidence.

Systematic Reviews of Disability and Rehabilitation Research available through NCDDR. Two other general registries are the Systematic Review Data Repository through the Agency for Healthcare Research and Quality (AHRQ) and the International Prospective Register of Systematic Reviews (Prospero), a collaborative of the University of York, Centre for Reviews and Dissemination, and the National Institutes of Health Research (UK National Health Service). The registries facilitate easy access to evidence-based knowledge generated through systematic reviews.

Professional/Trade Organizations

Many professional organizations have a repository of systematic reviews relevant to their particular specialty areas. In the area of rehabilitation there are several such groups (see **Table 1**) that provide best evidence in the form of systematic reviews and clinical guidelines.

Databases

The next source for locating systematic reviews is databases. **Table 1** provides information on common general databases (MEDLINE, CINAHL [Cumulative Index to Nursing and Allied Health Literature], and PsychInfo) as well as rehabilitation-focused databases such as PEDro, PsycBITE, OT Seeker, and speechBITE.

SYSTEMATIC REVIEWS AND CLINICAL GUIDELINES

Because systematic reviews pool and synthesize the evidence, they provide a more powerful and reliable conclusion that should underpin clinical practice guidelines (CPGs). Because systematic reviews typically cover narrow questions, multiple systematic reviews may form the evidence for the development of CPGs. The Institute of Medicine (IOM) states that CPGs are "statements that include recommendations intended to optimize patient care that are informed by a systematic review of evidence and an assessment of the benefits and harms of alternative care options."[9] To be trustworthy," guidelines should be based on a systematic evidence review, developed by a panel of multidisciplinary experts, provide a clear explanation of the logical relationships between alternative care options and health outcomes, and provide ratings of both the quality of evidence and the strength of the recommendations."[10] Sources to search for guidelines (see **Table 1**) include the National Guidelines Clearinghouse, the Scottish Intercollegiate Network, Guidelines International Network (G-I-N), as well as many professional medical organizations.

USING SYSTEMATIC REVIEWS: A CASE STUDY OF AN ELDERLY PATIENT WITH A HIP FRACTURE AND ACUTE DELIRIUM
Hip Fracture, Falls, and Delirium: The Background

Because the most common treatment of a fractured hip is surgery, admission to a hospital followed by a stay in rehabilitation puts elderly patients at risk for the development of acute delirium. In hospitalized patients with a hip fracture, the incidence of delirium is reported to be as high as 62%, with greater rates in those with preexisting psychiatric disorders, such as dementia, and those who are more than 65 years of age.[11] Delirium is the most frequent complication among postoperative patients with a hip fracture with symptoms occurring as early as the first postoperative day and persisting long after discharge from the acute care environment.[12] According to Cole and colleagues,[13] this situation, called persistent delirium, may contribute to worse outcomes (mortality, nursing home placement, decreased function, and altered cognition). Lee and colleagues[14] (http://www.mdconsult.com.libproxy2.umdnj.edu/das/article/body/ 441001859-2/jorg=clinics&source=&sp=26159544&sid=0/N/1156529/1.html?issn= 0030-5898 - r13000047036) performed a prospective cohort study of 232 elderly patients with hip fracture who were managed operatively. Delirium lasting longer than 4 weeks was associated with increased mortality at 2 years compared with patients with delirium lasting less than 4 weeks. Functional decline (ie, the ability to walk independently) was observed to be significant in this group.

Delirium, characterized by a fluctuating course of disturbances in orientation, memory, attention, thought, and behavior,[15] goes largely unrecognized by health care providers.[16,17] The exact mechanism for development of delirium is not known, but it is thought to be related to a cholinergic deficiency that impinges on the central nervous system.[18] Delirium can occur in 1 of 3 clinical forms (**Box 1**). A single factor rarely results in delirium, but instead delirium results from the interaction of environmental, procedural, and treatment factors.[15,19] Aspects of the physical environment, in which vulnerable patients are subjected to multiple changes in staff, disturbed sleep, discomfort, dehydration, and immobilization, are reported to be major precipitating factors for the onset of delirium.[20] Ski and O'Connell[21] noted that caring for patients with delirium is challenging not only for the management of their basic nursing care needs but also because they are prone to falls.

Case Study

PJ is a 72-year-old woman admitted to the rehabilitation setting following surgical repair of a fracture of the head of the femur 6 days ago. She is in a wheelchair. She is admitted to improve her ability to walk independently and without pain. Her son relates that her medical history involves hearing loss (she wears bilateral hearing aids, which were lost during her hospitalization), osteoarthritis, hypertension, and diabetes controlled with medication. She has smoked 1 pack of cigarettes a day for as long as he can remember. For the past 5 years since the death of her husband, she has been apathetic and withdrawn and experiencing insomnia, which has been difficult to treat. Current medications include hydrochlorothiazide (Diuril), glyburide (Micronase), alprazolam (Xanax), diazepam (Valium), and large quantities of aspirin for arthritic pain. The nurse learns that during her recent hospitalization the patient had an episode in which she saw her late husband and he was telling her to stop laying

Box 1 Types of delirium	
Type of Delirium	**Characteristics**
Hyperactive	Restlessness Hypervigilance Agitation Aggression Delusions Hallucinations
Hypoactive	Decreased psychomotor activity Lethargy Drowsiness Apathy Withdrawal
Mixed	A combination of the hyperactive and hypoactive types

around in bed and take control of her life. At present, the patient is paying no attention to the conversation between the admitting nurse and her son. She looks sleepy. When her son leaves, the nurse places her in bed in her private room and draws the blinds and turns out the light so that the patient can rest. Thirty minutes later, the nurse enters the room to find the patient lying on the floor, the telephone is beside her, and she is yelling at the facility telephone operator to call the police to get her out of this prison.

SYSTEMATIC REVIEWS AND ACUTE DELIRIUM

A search of the Cochrane Library for systematic review using the key words "delirium," "acute confusion," "elderly," "risk factors," "screening," and "prevention" yielded 2 reviews.[22,23] The first review[22] examined only the prevalence of delirium in medical patients and was excluded. The second[23] examined delirium prevention in the elderly in long-term care; however, it was an empty review and was also excluded. The search was then extended to include systematic reviews from the Joanna Briggs Library, which yielded 2 reviews.[24,25] Extending the search further to include MEDLINE over a 15-year period (1999–2014) provided an additional 10 systematic reviews for a total of 12 systematic reviews on acute delirium. In reviewing the abstracts of all studies to determine inclusion, only those focused on nonintensive or noncritical care patients and/or implications for surgical patients were selected for inclusion. Of the 12 selected for inclusion, 6 were focused on identifying risk factors, 2 on screening in the non–critically ill patient, and 4 on prevention. **Table 2** provides the characteristics of these reviews.

Identifying Risk Factors

In a review of 24 cohort studies with more than 1000 subjects, Mattar and Childs[24] reported that patients in different hospital settings showed different risk factors. For example, sepsis and alcohol use were the most significant risk factors among medical patients. Surgical patients, including those undergoing orthopedic surgery, were reported to be at risk for the development of acute delirium if they had high APACHE (Acute Physiology and Chronic Health Evaluation) II scores ($\geq$16) and multiple blood transfusions. The review also identified benzodiazepines (eg, Ativan) as the most significant drug associated with delirium in patients. Mattar and Childs[24] also reported several physiologic measures as being significantly associated with delirium, including low tryptophan levels, high plasma cortisol, high interleukin-6 levels, anemia, hypocalcemia, hyponatremia, azotemia, increased liver enzymes, hyperbilirubinemia, and metabolic acidosis.

Van Rampaey and colleagues[26] identified that 3 different doses of morphine influenced the onset of delirium. The highest odds ratio for development of delirium was related to an intermediate daily morphine dose of between 7.2 and 18.6 mg. Fong and colleagues[27] found that meperidine was consistently associated with an increased risk of postoperative delirium in elderly surgical patients.

In a review of 25 studies, Dasgupta and colleagues[28] reported that the incidence of delirium ranged from 5.1% to 52.2%, with higher rates found after hip fracture, simultaneous bilateral knee replacement, and aortic surgeries. Findings suggested that older age, functional and sensory impairment, depression, cognitive impairment, psychotropic drug use, and having more than 1 comorbidity were associated with postoperative delirium. In a review of 22 studies, Kahn and colleagues[29] similarly reported that age, cognitive impairment, depression, anticholinergic drugs, and lorazepam use were associated with an increased risk for the development of delirium.

Screening

Although delirium is typically diagnosed by psychiatric consultation using the Diagnostic and Statistical Manual of Mental Disorders, Fourth Edition (DSM-IV), screening tools such as the confusion assessment method (CAM) have been developed for use as an adjunct to more formal cognitive assessment. The CAM provides a 4-part algorithm for diagnosis of delirium: (1) an acute onset of fluctuating mental status change, (2) inattention, (3) disorganized thinking, and (4) an altered level of consciousness. The diagnosis of delirium is made if the patient presents with 1 and 2 and either 3 or 4.[30] In a systematic review by Wei and colleagues,[30] findings from 239 primary studies with a total of 1071 subjects were examined. Results indicated an overall sensitivity of 95% (range 46% to 100%) and specificity of 89% for the detection of delirium. Reasons for the low sensitivity rates were determined to be use of the CAM tool by those who were not trained in its use and the inclusion of populations that had a high rate of dementia and depression, which may have masked delirium. It was reported in this systematic review that patients identified with CAM had more serious falls, increased rates of mortality, adverse postsurgical outcomes (eg, sepsis), ineffective pain control, longer lengths of stay, an increase in the use of restraints, and greater instances of institutionalization after discharge. Mason and colleagues[31] reviewed 5 studies dealing with postoperative delirium and concluded that type and route of anesthesia had no effect on developing the condition.

Prevention

The 4 systematic reviews on the prevention of acute delirium organized interventions as pharmacologic, nonpharmacologic, or a combination.[25,32–34] An early systematic review by Cole and colleagues[32] found that geriatric consultation within 24 hours of hip surgery reduced the incidence and severity of delirium, and that preventive strategies worked better among surgical patients as opposed to medical patients. This systematic review reported that nursing interventions were as effective as physician interventions in preventing delirium.

Hempenius and colleagues[33] examined 8 RCTs on pharmacologic interventions and 8 studies on the use of nonpharmacologic interventions to determine whether the use of any intervention prevents delirium. The population of patients studied included surgical patients in the perioperative period undergoing cardiopulmonary bypass, gastric procedures, or orthopedic procedures. Preventive interventions included educating the nursing staff about delirium, using systematic cognitive screening, implementing geriatric consultative services, instituting a scheduled pain protocol in patients experiencing traumatic hip fracture surgery, psychiatric consultation before surgery, and daily supportive psychotherapy throughout the patient stay. Intravenous bolus or drip diazepam; flunitrazepam; and/or pethidine, gabapentin, donepezil, rivastigmine, and risperidone were evaluated versus placebo. The timing of the medications administered varied from before surgery to the first 3 nights after surgery. Findings indicated that effectiveness was similar for pharmacologic intervention only, single intervention, or multicomponent intervention.

Milisen and colleagues[34] synthesized the findings of 7 studies on interventions to prevent the development of delirium. The primary goal of the review was to identify the types and efficacy of multicomponent nonpharmacologic prevention strategies for delirium in hospitalized older adults. The review included a total of 1248 medical and surgical patients aged 65 years and older. Interventions included preoperative consultation or consultation within 24 hours after surgery and daily visits by a geriatrician or geriatric nurse specialist. The review concluded that strategies to prevent

Table 2
Systematic reviews on delirium

Citation	Characteristics	Major Findings
Cole[32]	This review comprises 10 clinical trials	Reorientation had greater effect in surgical patients. There was no difference in outcome for the prevention strategy related to provider (physician vs nurse)
Milisen et al,[34] 2005	This review comprises 7 studies of which 3 were RCTs, 3 controlled studies, and 1 before-after study	The 4 prevention studies involved the use of multidisciplinary protocols. Strategies to prevent delirium were more efficacious than strategies to treat delirium. Basic needs related to comfort, safety, hydration, and oxygenation proved to be the most effective strategies in preventing delirium. Surgical patients benefited most
Fong et al,[27] 2006	This review comprises 6 studies comparing different opioid analgesics on postoperative delirium and cognitive decline and 5 studies comparing intravenous and epidural routes of administering analgesia	Meperidine (Demerol) was consistently associated with an increased risk of delirium in elderly surgical patients
Dasgupta et al,[28] 2006	This review comprises 25 studies of which 21 were risk factor studies, 3 were validation studies only, and 1 was both a validation and risk factor study	Findings revealed that older age, cognitive impairment, functional and sensory impairment, depression, preoperative psychotropic drug use, institutional residence, and more than 1 comorbidity were associated with postoperative delirium
van Rampaey et al,[26] 2008	This review comprises 5 prospective cohort studies and 1 chart review	Intensive smoking, daily use of more than 3 units of alcohol, and living alone at home were environmental factors contributing to the development of delirium. In the domain of chronic disorders a preexisting cognitive impairment was an important risk factor. In the domain of factors related to acute illness the use of drains, tubes, and catheters; acute illness scores; the use of psychoactive medication; and a preceding period of sedation, coma, or mechanical ventilation showed significant risk. Environmental risk factors were isolation, the absence of visitors, the absence of visible daylight, a transfer from another ward, and the use of physical restraints

Wei et al,[30] 2008	This study comprises 239 original articles that include validation studies, adaptation studies, translation studies, and application studies. Validation studies evaluated performance of the CAM against a reference standard	The CAM has helped to improve identification of delirium in clinical settings. Training in the use of the tool is recommended
Hempenius et al,[33] 2011	This meta-analysis included 16 studies of which 9 were randomized controlled studies, 4 before-and-after studies, and 3 non–randomized controlled studies	The included studies showed a positive result of any intervention to prevent delirium. No specific intervention was identified as the best
Mason et al,[31] 2010	This review comprises 21 studies, 5 of which deal with postoperative delirium	There was no effect of anesthesia type on the odds ratio of developing postoperative delirium
Koster[38]	This review comprises 7 prospective cohort studies and 3 retrospective chart reviews	Cognitive impairment, older age, depression, and a history of stroke had higher odds ratios as predisposing factors to acute delirium following cardiac surgery
Mattar & Childs,[24] 2012	This review comprises 24 cohort studies. Of these 2 were retrospective and the remaining prospective observational studies	Risk factors for development of delirium differ by hospital unit. Benzodiazepines should be avoided as much as possible. Sepsis and alcohol, high APACHE scores, and older age were also identified
Kahn et al,[29] 2012	This review comprises 22 cohort studies	Age, cognitive impairment, depression, anticholinergic drugs, and lorazepam use were associated with an increased risk for developing delirium
Thomas et al,[25] in press	This review comprises 10 studies. Of these, 3 were randomized controlled studies, and the other 7 were prospective cohort or case-control studies	The effect of multicomponent interventions, compared with usual care, on the prevention of delirium was statistically significant. Patients who received multicomponent interventions had 31% lower risk of developing delirium. These interventions also lessened the duration and severity of delirium, although these findings were not statistically significant

Abbreviations: APACHE, Acute Physiology and Chronic Health Evaluation; CAM, confusion assessment method.

delirium were more efficacious than strategies to treat delirium. The prevention strategies included attention to basic needs, such as fluid/electrolyte balance, pain relief, adequate hydration and nutrition, bowel/bladder function, nutrition, and mobilization. In these patients, delirium was prevented in one-third of the group. A subgroup analysis revealed that surgical patients benefited most from any intervention. Multicomponent intervention was most effective for those experiencing specifically visual impairment or cognitive impairment.

Thomas and colleagues[25] synthesized the evidence from 10 studies on nonpharmacologic multicomponent interventions for prevention of delirium in hospitalized older adult patients not in intensive care. The effect of multicomponent interventions, compared with usual care, was statistically significant. Patients who received multicomponent interventions had 31% lower risk of developing delirium. These interventions also lessened the duration and severity of delirium, although these findings were not statistically significant. Typical nonpharmacologic multicomponent interventions included the use of specialized clinical staff/volunteers, geriatric/psychiatric consultation, staff education, patient orientation, addressing visual and hearing needs, sleep enhancement, medication review, hydration and nutrition, early mobilization, pain management, addressing bowel and bladder functions, and prevention and treatment of medical complications. These interventions were performed by a variety of individuals including unit staff (nurses, physicians, assistants), elder life specialists, volunteers, and family members.

SYSTEMATIC REVIEW DATA APPLIED TO THE CASE STUDY

Preventing delirium is the responsibility of all rehabilitation professionals working with older adults. Reducing or eliminating risk factors begins with early identification and treatment. Because there is no pharmacologic treatment for delirium, the rehabilitation team must work together to create an environment in which the confused patient has the potential to recover.[35,36]

Following a review of systematic reviews and evidence-based guidelines for the prevention and management of delirium in postoperative patients with a hip fracture, Holly and colleagues[37] developed audit criteria that can be used to evaluate care in this case study. Five audit criteria were proposed that capture key clinical recommendations emerging from the systematic review data[1]: "All elderly patients with a hip fracture are assessed for risk factors for developing delirium daily using a valid and reliable tool[2]; the environment of the patient with hip fracture is assessed daily for conduciveness to maintaining sensory orientation[3]; all patients with hip fracture receive essential nursing care[4]; appropriate clinical criteria are applied to confirm a diagnosis of delirium in patients with hip fracture[5]; and nonpharmacologic interventions are employed before pharmacologic interventions in patients with hip fracture with a diagnosis of delirium (p27)". The first 3 of these criteria are relevant to the case study at hand. Criteria 4 and 5 would follow accomplishment of the first 3 criteria.

Table 3 takes the audit criteria and systematic review data and suggests care that should have been implemented in this case. The standards for prevention and management of delirium in clients with a hip fracture were not met in this case. Criterion 1 reinforces the need for assessment for delirium at least daily. Given the fluctuating nature of acute delirium and the patient's history of mixed delirium, daily assessment (an assessment on admission) was vital for early detection and management. Use of a valid and reliable tool, such as the CAM, is important. Had assessment for delirium been done on admission it is likely that the multiple risk factors for delirium would

Table 3
Systematic review findings applied to case study (PJ)

	Data	Care Evaluation and Recommendation
Criterion 1: assess for risk factors for developing delirium daily using a valid and reliable tool	Risk factors identified on systematic review present in case study include: • Older age • Hip fracture • High-risk medications: valium, Xanax • Polypharmacy • Hyperactive delirium while in hospital • Sensory impairment: hearing loss • >1 comorbidity • Cognitive impairment • Delusions in hospital • Possible dehydration from a diuretic	• No indication that risk factors were assessed. • No evidence of cognitive assessment • No instrument was used to screen for delirium Screening for delirium should have been done immediately on admission. PJ presented with signs of hypoactive delirium and safety measures needed to be instituted
Criterion 2: the environment of the patient with hip fracture is assessed daily for conduciveness to maintaining sensory orientation	Patient is placed in bed with blinds drawn and lights turned out so that she can rest	No evidence that sensory impairment was assessed The environment is not conducive to maintaining sensory orientation. PJ has hearing loss and is now in a new environment with little visual stimulation
Criterion 3: all patients with hip fracture receive essential nursing care	Essential care includes promoting safety, comfort, hydration, oxygenation, and adequate pain relief	No assessment was made of gait in order to determine safety needs No evidence of orientation to new environment No evidence of toileting before placing patient in bed There needs to be a comprehensive assessment of safety and physiologic needs

have been noted and that it would have been recognized that PJ was presenting with signs of hypoactive delirium (decreased psychomotor activity, lethargy, drowsiness, apathy, withdrawal). Criterion 2 addresses the environment and the need to maintain sensory orientation. PJ had a known hearing impairment with loss of her hearing aids while in the hospital. She was then placed in a new environment without orientation and the room was darkened, imposing additional visual impairment. The final criterion relevant to this case, that essential nursing care be administered, also showed a deficit. PJ's safety needs regarding ambulation were not assessed and general toileting was not done before leaving her in a darkened room.

Delirium is a frequently occurring syndrome in postoperative patients with a hip fracture. However, it often goes unrecognized, resulting in functional decline, increased hospital length of stay, prolonged recovery, hospital readmission, increased health care cost, and mortality. In addition, standardized approaches to improve the care of postoperative patients with delirium are not routinely followed.[37] By using up-to-date evidence, the nurse may be able to alter the circumstances leading to delirium as well as decreasing the possibility of falls.

SUMMARY

Practicing evidence-based rehabilitation requires clinicians to understand how evidence fits into the decision-making process along with patient preference, clinical expertise, and clinical context. Knowing how to search for the best available evidence in the form of systematic reviews and CPGs that are based on systematic reviews is a critical skill. Using a systematic search approach is more effective and time efficient. Drawing on the results of systematic reviews, it is possible to make recommendations for clinical practice that can be implemented and tested.

REFERENCES

1. Holly C, Salmond S, Saimbert MK. Comprehensive systematic review for advanced nursing practice. New York: Springer; 2012.
2. Dijkers MP, Bushnik T, Heinemann AW, et al. Systematic reviews for informing rehabilitation practice: an introduction. Arch Phys Med Rehabil 2012;93: 912–8.
3. IOM (Institute of Medicine). Clinical practice guidelines we can trust. Washington, DC: The National Academies Press; 2011.
4. IOM (Institute of Medicine). Finding what works in health care: standards for systematic reviews. Washington, DC: The National Academies Press; 2011.
5. Wieland LS, Skoetz N, Manheimer E, et al. Yoga treatment for chronic non-specific low-back pain. Cochrane Database of Systematic Reviews 2013.
6. Cramer H, Lauche R, Dobos G. A systematic review and meta-analysis of yoga for low back pain. Clin J Pain 2013;29(5):450–60.
7. Salmond SW. Finding the evidence to support evidence-based practice. Orthop Nurs 2013;32(1):16–24.
8. Schlosser RW, Sigaffos J. 'Empty' reviews and evidence-based practice. Evid Based Commun Assess Interv 2009;3:1–3.
9. Consensus report, Institute of Medicine. Clinical practice guidelines we can trust. 2011. Available at: http://www.iom.edu/Reports/2011/Clinical-Practice-Guidelines-We-Can-Trust.aspx. Accessed March 18, 2013.
10. NHLBI. About systematic evidence reviews and clinical practice guidelines. Available at: http://www.nhlbi.nih.gov/guidelines/about.htm#contents. Accessed March 18, 2013.
11. Robertson BD, Robertson TJ. Postoperative delirium after hip fracture. J Bone Joint Surg Am 2006;88(9):2060–8.
12. Kzyirids TC. Post-operative delirium after hip fracture treatment: a review of the current literature. Psychosoc Med 2006;3:1–12.
13. Cole MG, Ciampi A, Belzile E, et al. Persistent delirium in older hospital patients: a systematic review of frequency and prognosis. Age Ageing 2009;38(1):19–26.
14. Lee KH, Ha YC, Lee YK, et al. Frequency, risk factors, and prognosis of prolonged delirium in elderly patients after hip fracture surgery. Clin Orthop Relat Res 2011; 469:2612–20.
15. Inouye SK. Current concepts: delirium in older persons. N Engl J Med 2006; 354(11):1157–65.
16. Inouye SK, Schlesinger MJ, Lydon TJ. Delirium: a symptom of how hospital care is failing older persons and a window to improve quality of hospital care. Am J Med 1999;106(5):565–73.

17. Steis MR, Fick DM. Are nurses recognizing delirium? A systematic review. J Gerontol Nurs 2008;34(9):40–8.
18. Holly C, Cantwell ER, Jadotte Y. Acute delirium: differentiation and care. Crit Care Nurs Clin North Am 2012;24(1):131–47.
19. Ljubisavljevic V, Kelly B. Risk factors for development of delirium among oncology patients. Gen Hosp Psychiatry 2003;25(5):345–52.
20. McCusker J, Cole MG, Dendukuri N, et al. Does delirium increase hospital stay? J Am Geriatr Soc 2003;51(11):1539.
21. Ski C, O'Connell B. Mismanagement of delirium places patients at risk. Aust J Adv Nurs 2006;23(3):42–6.
22. Siddiqi N, Holt R, Britton AM, et al. Interventions for preventing delirium in hospitalised patients. Cochrane Database Syst Rev 2007;(2):CD005563. http://dx.doi.org/10.1002/14651858.CD005563.pub2.
23. Clegg A, Siddiqi N, Heaven A, et al. Interventions for preventing delirium in older people in institutional long-term care. Cochrane Database Syst Rev 2014;(1):CD009537.
24. Mattar C, Childs CI. Factors causing acute delirium in critically ill adult patients: a systematic review. JBI Database of Systematic Reviews and Implementation Reports JBI000464 2012;10(3):187–231.
25. Thomas E, Smith JE, Forrester DA, et al. The effectiveness of non-pharmacological multi-component interventions for the prevention of delirium in non-intensive care unit older adult hospitalized patients: a systematic review protocol. JBI Database of Systematic Reviews & Implementation Reports 2013;11(7):361–74.
26. Van Rampaey B, Schuurmansc MJ, Shortridge-Baggett LM, et al. Risk factors for intensive care delirium: a systematic review. Intensive Crit Care Nurs 2008;24:98–107.
27. Fong HK, Sands L, Leung J. The role of postoperative analgesia in delirium and cognitive decline in elderly patients: a systematic review. Anesth Analg 2006;102:1255–66.
28. Dasgupta M, Dumbrell AC, Maw J. Preoperative risk assessment for delirium after noncardiac surgery: a systematic review. J Am Geriatr Soc 2006;54:1578–89.
29. Kahn BA, Zawahiri M, Campbell NL, et al. Delirium in hospitalized patients: implications of current evidence on clinical practice and future avenues for research-a systematic evidence review. J Hosp Med 2012;7(7):580–9.
30. Wei LA, Wei BA, Fearing MA, et al. The confusion assessment method: a systematic review of current usage. J Am Geriatr Soc 2008;56:823–30.
31. Mason S, Storr AN, Ritcheia G. Post operative cognitive dysfunction and post operative delirium: a systematic review with metaanalysis. J Alzheimers Dis 2010;22:S67–79.
32. Cole MG, Primeau F, McCusker J. Effectiveness of interventions to prevent delirium in hospitalized patients: a systematic review. Can Med Assoc J 1996;155(9):1263–8.
33. Hempenius L, van Leeuwen B, van Asselt D, et al. Structured analyses of interventions to prevent delirium. Int J Geriatr Psychiatry 2011;26:441–50.
34. Milisen K, Lemiengre J, Braes T, et al. Multicomponent intervention strategies for managing delirium in hospitalized older people: a systematic review. J Adv Nurs 2005;52(1):79–90.
35. Huber G. Prevention and management of delirium in geriatric rehabilitation. Top Geriatr Rehabil 2012;28(3):148–56.
36. Babin KA, Miley H. Implementing the best available evidence in early delirium identification in elderly hip surgery patients. Int J Evid Based Healthc 2013;11:39–45.

37. Holly C, Rittenmeyer L, Weeks SM. Evidence-based clinical audit criteria for the prevention and management of delirium in the postoperative patient with a hip fracture. Orthop Nurs 2014;33(1):27–34.

38. Koster S, Hensen AG, Schuurmans MJ, et al. Risk factors of delirium after cardiac surgery: a systematic review. Eur J Cardiovasc Nurs 2011;10(4):197–204.

Evidence in Mental Health

Susan Mace Weeks, DNP, RN, CNS, LMFT[a,b,*]

KEYWORDS

- Systematic review • Evidence synthesis • Mental health • Mental illness
- Evidence-based health care

KEY POINTS

- Mental health practitioners should use synthesized evidence as the basis of their clinical decision making.
- Systematic reviews are a credible source of synthesized evidence.
- Standards developed and refined by credible organizations should be used when conducting systematic reviews.

INTRODUCTION

Health practitioners wishing to positively improve health outcomes for the clients they serve have access to a unique set of collated tools to guide their practice. Systematic reviews provide guidance in the form of synthesized evidence that can form the basis of decision making as they provide care for their clients. Whether the clients being served are individuals, families, groups, or communities, systematic reviews provide a unique foundation of guidance on which clinical decisions can be made.

WHAT IS A SYSTEMATIC REVIEW?

A systematic review is a document that describes a scientific process used to collate individual research studies, or other forms of evidence, into a useful format to guide practitioners' decision making. Scholars conducting a systematic review use standards and guidelines developed by reputable organizations to systematically synthesize varied forms of evidence in a transparent and reproducible manner. Organizations providing standards and guidelines for the development of systematic reviews include the Joanna Briggs Institute (http://joannabriggs.org/), the Cochrane Collaboration (http://www.cochrane.org/), the Campbell Collaboration (http://www.campbellcollaboration.org/),

Disclosure: None.
[a] Texas Christian University – Harris College of Nursing and Health Sciences, TCU Box 298620, Fort Worth, TX 76129, USA; [b] Harris College of Nursing and Health Sciences, TCU Center for Evidence Based Practice and Research: A Collaborating Center of the Joanna Briggs Institute, Fort Worth, TX 79129, USA
* Texas Christian University – Harris College of Nursing and Health Sciences, TCU Box 298620, Fort Worth, TX 76129.
E-mail address: s.weeks@tcu.edu

Nurs Clin N Am 49 (2014) 525–531
http://dx.doi.org/10.1016/j.cnur.2014.08.007
nursing.theclinics.com
0029-6465/14/$ – see front matter © 2014 Elsevier Inc. All rights reserved.

and the Institute of Medicine (http://www.iom.edu/Reports/2011/Finding-What-Works-in-Health-Care-Standards-for-Systematic-Reviews/Standards.aspx).

PROCESS OF SYSTEMATIC REVIEW

The process of producing a systematic review begins with asking a well-formed clinical question. Questions emerge frequently in the minds of practitioners as they seek to provide excellent care to clients in hopes of producing positive outcomes. Often the clinical question starts as a vague sense of wondering if there might be a better option for a given client or situation. The systematic reviewer translates that sense of clinical unease into a format that can be answered through the systematic review process.

The clinical question is often expressed in a "PICO" or "PICOT" format. The aspects of a "PICO" or "PICOT" question are as follows:

Population: What is the specific type of client(s)?
Intervention: What option for treatment do you wish to explore?
Comparator: What would the treatment be if you were not exploring the intervention?
Outcomes: How can you measure if clinical improvement has been achieved?
Time: Within what time frame would you expect to see improvement?

An example of a clinical question expressed in the PICOT format is: What is the effectiveness of group therapy, as compared with individual therapy, on 6-month medication compliance rates for individuals dealing with a new diagnosis of schizophrenia? This same question with labels identified for the PICOT elements is: What is the effectiveness of group therapy (intervention), as compared with individual therapy (comparator), on 6-month (time) medication compliance rates (outcome) for individuals dealing with a new diagnosis of schizophrenia (population)?

The PICO or PICOT formats are useful when asking questions best answered by quantitative evidence, such as randomized controlled trials or other experimental research designs. Other clinical questions, particularly those dealing with experience or meaning, are better answered by evidence from qualitative literature. When the question being asked is best addressed by qualitative evidence, a "PIC" format is suggested. The aspects of a "PIC" question include:

Population: What is the specific type of client(s)?
Phenomenon of Interest: What is the experience or condition of focus?
Context: What is the situation in which the experience or condition occurs?

An example of a clinical question expressed in the PIC format is: What is the experience of individuals with a diagnosis of schizophrenia dealing with marginalization in the workplace? This same question with labels identified for the PIC elements is: What is the experience of individuals with a diagnosis of schizophrenia (population) dealing with marginalization (phenomenon of interest) in the workplace (context)?

Following the formation of an answerable clinical question the systematic reviewer begins to proceed down a structured path that is, as one might guess, quite systematic. Sequential steps of articulating the inclusion and exclusion criteria for the type of evidence to be retrieved are outlined. The strategy used to search for the best evidence is described. The description includes a list of the databases searched, how gray (unpublished) literature was sought, key words used for the search, and any additional levels of searching. Additional levels of searching include searching for the key words of the articles obtained through the first-level search, and searching the reference lists of the articles retrieved from the prior two levels of searching. The reviewer may also hand-search the table of contents of the journals most often represented in the retrieved search results.

Following the search process, retrieved articles are critically appraised to determine their quality. Those studies and/or articles judged to be of high quality are included in the systematic review. Those studies and/or articles judged to be of poor quality are excluded following a notation of the rationale for exclusion. The systematic reviewers must make a judgment call for studies and/or articles that are not clearly of high quality or clearly of poor quality. If there is disagreement among the review team regarding the quality of a study and/or article, the reviewers discuss and debate the quality of the source until agreement is reached. The articles that pass the phase of critical appraisal are then synthesized in a quantitative manner, such as in a meta-analysis graph, or in a qualitative manner, such as through a meta-aggregation.

Following the synthesis of the evidence, guidance for practice implications is developed to inform health practitioners functioning at the point of care. Additional implications, such as those for research and/or education, may also be developed. The systematic review is then made available through publication or other forms of scholarly dissemination.

A logical question to follow the previous description of a systematic review is, "Why?" Why would it matter if we knew the exact way to treat something that may not have relevance or applicability? The reason is because evidence does matter. Evidence matters when you are dealing with a new mother who may be fearful to hold her baby for the first time. Evidence matters when a family member receives a health diagnosis that will change the course of their life. Evidence matters to an individual with a chronic health condition struggling with symptom management. In short, evidence matters for all health conditions (**Fig. 1**).[1]

SYSTEMATIC REVIEWS FOR MENTAL HEALTH PRACTITIONERS

Individuals dealing with a mental health challenge have significant barriers to overcome as they struggle with the implications of their illness. Likewise, mental health clinicians have significant challenges as they seek credible evidence to guide their decision making. Fortunately, there is an emerging body of literature that has been synthesized in the form of systematic reviews to guide mental health practitioners.

Although multiple organizations produce and maintain systematic reviews relevant to mental health practitioners, only one of those organizations provides both systematic reviews and other varied forms of clinical guidance based on systematic reviews. The Joanna Briggs Institute, founded in 1996, is the global leader in the synthesis and dissemination of varied forms of synthesized evidence. In addition to systematic reviews, the Joanna Brigs Institute also provides evidence summaries, which are a condensed version of a systematic review. Additional forms of evidence based on the results of systematic reviews are also available from the Joanna Briggs Institute. Those forms of evidence include

- Practice manual: more than 600 policies and procedures to guide health practitioners delivering care based on the best available evidence
- Best practice information sheets: short version of critical "need to know" information for health practitioners
- Consumer information sheets: information designed for health care consumers
- Systematic review protocols: plan to be followed for systematic review in progress
- Titles of proposed systematic reviews: title and PICO/PICOT/PIC question elements for proposed systematic reviews

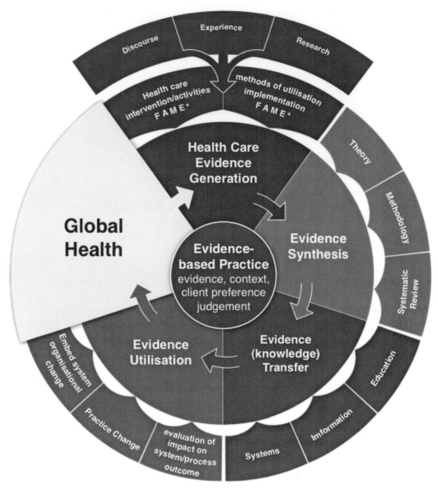

Fig. 1. The Joanna Briggs Institute Model of Evidence-Based Healthcare. FAME, feasibility, appropriateness, meaningfulness, and effectiveness. (*Courtesy of* the Joanna Briggs Institute, The University of Adelaide, South Australia, Australia; with permission.)

- Quality improvement clinical audit criteria
- Clinical outcomes tracking tools to evaluate the impact of care

Systematic reviews with relevance for mental health practitioners represent a wide variety of topics. Systematic reviews are available for various mental health diagnoses, such as schizophrenia as seen in a systematic review on supportive therapies for schizophrenia.[2] The varied populations served by mental health practitioners including children, older adults, and individuals with chronic mental illness are represented in available systematic reviews, such as a review on enhancing the well-being of postpartum women.[3] Treatment modalities including telemental health, community mental health, and shared decision-making strategies used to care for individuals with mental health challenges have been evaluated in completed systematic reviews. One example is a systematic review on the effectiveness of individual and group therapy.[4] Issues of risk for mental health clients and practitioners including aggression, violence, and fall prevention have been explored through systematic reviews, such as a systematic review on fall prevention among adult psychiatric patients.[5] Existing systematic reviews explore a variety of other issues including mental health care settings,[6] self-care for various mental health diagnoses,[7] education for mental health consumers,[8] and mental health policy issues.[9]

SAMPLE MENTAL HEALTH SYSTEMATIC REVIEW

To illustrate the value of a systematic review conducted on a mental health topic, a recently published systematic review was evaluated. The selected systematic review addresses the experiences of family members caring for an individual with schizophrenia.[10] The value of this systematic review is summarized in the following list:

- Unique aspects of this systematic review: This review synthesized qualitative evidence (evidence of meaningfulness) and was conducted by an international review team. The language skills of the review team allowed the inclusion of studies in the English and Thai languages.
- Potential usefulness of this systematic review: This review could be used to develop clinical interventions, programming for patients and/or their caregivers, policy briefs, and recommendations for future research.
- Implications for practice: The results of this systematic review lead to suggestions to partner with family members, be aware of caregiver responses, provide information to caregivers, and train caregivers who will be caring for individuals with schizophrenia.
- Possible methods to assess the outcomes for the practice changes suggested by this systematic review: Outcomes to be considered could include clinical outcomes of patients and/or their caregivers, patient compliance, caregiver compliance, participation of patients and/or caregivers, rating scales of caregiver experiences, and quality-of-life scales.
- Potential tools based on this systematic review: Other practice tools that could be developed from this systematic review include an evidence summary, best practice information sheets for clinicians, consumer information sheets, quality improvement clinical audit criteria, clinical outcomes tracking tools, and suggested policies and procedures for supporting individuals caring for those with schizophrenia.
- Policy implications: Guidance for community programming to support caregivers of individuals with schizophrenia could be drawn from this systematic review.
- Implications for future research: This systematic review concludes that future research should focus on testing caregiver intervention programs, identifying best practice guidelines, and conducting further metasynthesis of this topic.
- Implications for education: Although not clearly stated in this systematic review, the results of the review suggest that content on the experiences of caregivers of individuals with schizophrenia should be included in the curricula of health professionals who will be interacting with and impacting this population. This would include health professions students, community health workers, and policy makers.

MENTAL HEALTH SYSTEMATIC REVIEW GAPS

Although there are existing systematic reviews available on a wide variety of topics, gaps in the body of mental health literature that has been synthesized by systematic review methodologies remain. Current gaps in systematic reviews on mental health topics include limited systematic reviews on

- Theories of mental health and mental illness
- Biologic and/or genetic basis of mental illness
- Cultural, legal, and ethical dimensions of mental illness and the treatment of mental illness
- Impact of health maintenance factors (eg, sleep, nutrition, exercise) on mental health and mental illness
- Complementary and alternative medicine strategies to support mental health and/or treat mental illness

EMERGING TOPICS FOR MENTAL HEALTH SYSTEMATIC REVIEWS

Topics of emerging significance for mental health practitioners should form the basis for future systematic reviews. These topics include interprofessional care modalities; public engagement in mental health care improvements; economic impact of mental health care including cost-benefit and cost-effectiveness analysis; and strategies to translate, implement, and evaluate knowledge related to mental health and mental illness. These topics are of increasing significance in mental health literature, and as their appearance in the professional literature increases, adequate bodies of evidence will be developed to warrant future systematic reviews.

SUMMARY

Health care evidence is generated based on an assessment of global health needs; however, without evidence synthesis the knowledge that has been generated through research cannot be transferred into the clinical setting. Knowledge must be translated, used, and evaluated in the clinical setting to positively impact global health. Without solid evidence synthesis the goal of improving health through health care practice based on sound evidence will not be realized.

Mental health professionals face significant challenges in dealing with a population that does not always seek or appreciate treatment. In addition, the lack of understanding of mental health treatment strategies by the population as a whole creates additional barriers. Funding and other resources to support mental health treatment are often limited. The challenges posed by limited resources make the role of systematic reviews even more significant. If mental health professionals wish to improve mental health on a global scale, they must have solid evidence in the form of systematic reviews on which they can base their treatment strategies.

REFERENCES

1. Pearson A, Weeks S, Stern C. Translation science and the JBI Model of Evidence-Based Healthcare. Philadelphia: Lippincott Williams & Wilkins; 2011.
2. Buckley LA, Pettit TA, Adams CE. Supportive therapy for schizophrenia. Cochrane Database Syst Rev 2007;(3):CD004716. Systematic Reviews.
3. Ni PK, Lin SK. The role of family and friends in providing social support towards enhancing the wellbeing of postpartum women: a comprehensive systematic review. JBI Library of Systematic Reviews 2011;9(10):313–70. Systematic Reviews.
4. Lockwood C, Page T, Conroy-Hiller T. Effectiveness of individual therapy and group therapy in the treatment of schizophrenia. Int J Evid Based Healthc 2004;2(10):309–38. Systematic Reviews.
5. Xu C, Tan X, Loh H, et al. Effectiveness of interventions for the assessment and prevention of falls in adult psychiatric patients: a systematic review. JBI Library of Systematic Reviews 2012;10(9):513–73. Systematic Reviews.

6. Norton-Westwood D, Pearson A, Robertson-Malt S. The ability of environmental healthcare design strategies to impact event related anxiety in pediatric patients: a comprehensive systematic review. JBI Library of Systematic Reviews 2011; 9(44):1828–82. Systematic Reviews.
7. Perkins SS, Murphy RR, Schmidt UU, et al. Self-help and guided self-help for eating disorders. Cochrane Database Syst Rev 2006;(3):CD004191. Systematic Reviews.
8. Griffiths RD, Fernandez RS, Mostacchi MS, et al. Comparison of educational interventions for mental health consumers receiving psychotropic medication. Int J Evid Based Healthc 2004;2(1):1–44. Systematic Reviews.
9. Murray J, Farrington DP, Sekol I, et al. Effects of parental imprisonment on child antisocial behavior and mental health: a systematic review. Campbell Systematic Reviews; 2009. p. 4. Systematic Reviews.
10. Tungpunkom P, Napa W, Chaniang S, et al. Caregiving experiences of families living with persons with schizophrenia: a systematic review. JBI Library of Systematic Reviews & Implementation Reports 2013;11(8):415–564.

Evidence in Public Health
Steps to Make It Real

Cassia Baldini Soares, RN, MPH, PhD[a],*, Tatiana Yonekura, RN, MSc (Nursing)[b],*,
Celia Maria Sivalli Campos, RN, MSc (Nursing), PhD[a],
Mabel Fernandes Figueiro, Bachelor (Library Sciences)[c]

KEYWORDS

- Literature review • Public health • Methodological studies
- Social determinants of health • Health impact assessment

KEY POINTS

- Effectiveness in public health entails establishing interventions that focus on the determinants of the health-disease process.
- The examination of the Cochrane Public Health Group reviews indicates trends in this direction, as well as the influence of the World Health Organization's Commission on Social Determinants of Health.
- Successful experiences, qualitative studies, reports, case studies, or other nonrandomized methodological designs should be taken as health evidence, based on narrative syntheses that show the impact on health determinants.
- Most of the public health reviews that were examined in this study deemed that the evidence was weak, moderate, or nonexistent.
- We identified that evidence of the analyzed public health interventions had some impact on health, as well as a difficulty in capturing the impact of their use.

INTRODUCTION

Public health problems are diversified, complex, and reflect the unequal distribution of wealth. Although it is a challenge to obtain evidence in public health, researchers can currently rely on theoretic and methodological frameworks as well as practical experiences to develop the synthesis of evidence.[1] Along with the growing governmental

Funding Sources: None.
Conflicts of Interests: None.
[a] Department of Collective Health Nursing, School of Nursing, University of São Paulo, Av. Dr. Enéas de Carvalho Aguiar 419, 2o. andar, São Paulo CEP 05403-000, Brazil; [b] The Nursing Graduate Program (PPGE), School of Nursing, University of São Paulo, Av. Dr. Enéas de Carvalho Aguiar 419, 2o. andar, São Paulo CEP 05403-000, Brazil; [c] Center of Health Technology Assessment, Hospital do Coração/HCor, Rua Abílio Soares, 250, 11° andar, Paraiso, São Paulo CEP 04005-002, Brazil
* Corresponding authors.
E-mail addresses: cassiaso@usp.br; tatyonekura@gmail.com

recognition of the importance of evidence-based public health, these resources are intended to lead the transformation of public health policies and practices toward equity.[1]

The systematic review (SR) indexed in the Cochrane Library as reviews of public health interest correspond with approximately half of the titles, with high diversity observed with regard to the interventions of interest (pharmacologic or nonpharmacologic), breadth of the context (local or national, home, community, work-related, or environmental), and object of the intervention (age group; cultural group; life cycle stage; other affinities/identities/demographic characteristics, such as gender, social class). This quantitative contingent is consistent with the current popularity of SR and evidence in public health and social sciences.[2]

Cochrane has adopted the reviewing of global public health issues, in compliance with the priorities of the Commission on Social Determinants of Health (CSDH) created in 2005[3] by the World Health Organization, as a support to address the social causes of health inequalities. The CSDH gathers and analyzes evidence about interventions that promote the reduction of health inequalities, focusing on the "causes of the causes" associated with the need to (1) improve living conditions; (2) address inequalities in the distribution of power, money, and resources; (3) measure and understand the problem, and (4) assess the impact of actions and interventions.[4]

The Cochrane Public Health Group (CPHG), in accordance with the Cochrane Health Equity Field, recommends that reviewers endeavor to analyze the effects of interventions on health equity,[5] which means addressing the theoretic and methodological challenges of exposing social determinants that generate inequalities.[4]

Traditional research designs tend to capture fragments of the well-established relationship between working and living conditions and the state of health or disease, which makes it difficult to clearly show the "causes of the causes." To clearly show the social determinants of health it is necessary to show the objects of intervention in their multiple determinations, thus exposing the mediatory connections between social structures and health problems. To show these requires research designs, such as case studies, and sources of evidence, such as experiences of health workers and of institutions that study failure and success rates, in addition to the research designs already used to measure the effectiveness of clinical treatments.[6]

This article therefore (1) discusses different views on the adequacy of synthesis of evidence methodologies for reviews in public health, and (2) examines the reviews registered in the CPHG to exemplify syntheses of evidence in public health and their applications and practical impacts.

METHODOLOGIES FOR SYNTHESIS OF EVIDENCE IN PUBLIC HEALTH: SOME CONTROVERSIES

Health literature reviews are based on systematization, analysis, and evaluation of primary research that places importance on research designs from the positivist tradition, with the potential to show hypotheses related to objects of the natural sciences. In this tradition, health literature reviews can be either based on biomedical categories or on the already existing health problems and/or on the associated risk factors,[7] with restrictions of the reviews and studies shaped by this paradigm being criticized by Marxism,[8] among other schools of thought.

A broad definition is appropriate:

Evidence-based public health is the process involved in providing the best available evidence to influence decisions about the effectiveness of policies and interventions and secure improvements in health and reduction in healthinequalities[1(p22)]

Researchers who take evidence-based public health into account should be familiar with the criticisms of the traditional premises that underlie the field, and should consider that the effectiveness of interventions on health determinants lies in broader social issues involving the working and living conditions of different social groups. The term "effectiveness" originated in the clinical sphere, in which it is generally used to evaluate a particular intervention. However, in public health, interventions involve multiple actions, usually determined by specific policies and programs.[9]

The number of studies on the effectiveness of interventions in public health is lower than of randomized clinical trials, largely because these investigations have complex methodological designs, usually stem from government programs, and therefore are often already underway.[9]

The most widespread criticism of these studies concerns the sources and the hierarchy of evidence. SRs with meta-analysis are the best sources of evidence for questions related to clinical interventions.[10] However, complex and interdisciplinary questions related to interventions in public health can also be answered using other sources of evidence, such as case reports or qualitative research.[11] These sources are increasingly being incorporated into the synthesis of evidence, because they bring the experience of those involved in the intervention and make it possible to deepen the knowledge about real-life situations.[6]

Although their synthesis constitutes a challenge, the results of observational studies used in public health[2] can be considered evidence.[12] These results cannot always be confirmed through randomized clinical trials, but this does not detract from their validity; they represent studies of a different nature that are methodologically consistent with their questions and objectives.[6] Unlike clinical trials, which evaluate changes in controlled variables through an intervention, observational studies are difficult to transform into variables.[6]

Successful interventions can come from sources other than reviews, resulting from the application of various tools, such as the Health Impact Assessment, developed to support the implementation of interventions in public health.[6]

There are divergences in public health in relation to the place assigned to evidence in health care, which is often considered a panacea.[8] The closer the theoretic-political perspective of the social determination to the health-disease process, the more public health departs from the premise that evidence has a universal and apolitical character, capable of repairing the course of health care. Evidence in health is a crucial instrument in the health production process, capable of guiding health workers in making decisions, similarly to clinical (and amplified clinical), epidemiology (and critical epidemiology), and health education (and emancipatory education). As such, it is not exempt from the different interests that underlie this process.[8]

SYSTEMATIC REVIEWS IN PUBLIC HEALTH: SOME RECOMMENDATIONS

With steps similar to those of other SRs, public health SRs should also be based on specific recommendations, such as those proposed by Bambra.[2]

They should be based on broad research questions. Public health programs and policies usually comprise sets of interventions, not just 1 specific intervention. Thus, it is recommended (1) to start with a scoping review to map the interventions of interest and to assist in the search strategies; (2) to verify the interventions among the proposals for public health programs and policies; and (3) to consider the appropriateness of evaluating them in separate questions.[2]

They should be performed by a team of specialists. Search strategy specialists can locate studies from specific areas with greater precision, and specialists in the object of study can help find studies in sources of gray and specialized literature.[2]

They should balance the optimal breadth of the search with the resources available, as well as the knowledge about the subject. A pilot study could be useful for recognizing where the studies are allocated and whether the search needs to be limited to more productive resources in the area and resources that are more consistent with the social situation to which the object of the review refers.[2]

They should also (1) use broad inclusion criteria, (2) encompass observational and qualitative research designs, (3) map the available studies about the intervention, and (4) establish a standard related to the reality of the studies available in the area. Once the team has discussed these parameters, the works that show good quality in each type of study included should be considered as evidence, and may include, depending on what is being studied, research designs not well situated in the hierarchy of evidence. Mapping the studies means understanding that the best evidence may not be available for the intervention of interest.[2]

It is advisable to use or adapt tools that are approved and available in the literature for data extraction and evaluation of studies by centers of excellence in reviews, or by similar reviews.[2]

Also, public health reviews should add narrative synthesis, which translates quantitative results into words, to the search for evidence in public health.[3] A qualitative meta-synthesis is a strategy recognized by Cochrane and recommended by its Qualitative Research Group to address the challenge of answering public health questions, which are explicative[13] and complex.[3]

The Joanna Briggs Institute (JBI) shows leadership in developing more inclusive methodologies such as meta-aggregation, which summarizes findings from qualitative studies. The JBI has also built methodology for synthesizing economic evidence and evidence from texts published by experts and health institutions. More recently, the institute developed guidelines for the development of mixed-method SRs. All these reviews are potentially relevant for public health because they make best use of results from different sources and the capacity of these results to instruct policy makers.[14]

CASE EXAMPLES OF REVIEWS IN PUBLIC HEALTH, AND THEIR IMPACT ON HEALTH AND USE

The CPHG supports, edits, and publishes SRs related to the effects of interventions on social determinants, with the goal of improving the health of the population.[5] There are currently (as of January, 2014) 9 finalized SRs registered in this group.

Among the examined examples of reviews is the search for evidence of objects amplified in their intervention components of interest and subject, broadening the unit that encompasses the object (from individual to population and from health problems to social determinants). These populations are considered heterogeneous, composed by different social groups, in terms of social characteristics, gender, ethnicity, and so forth. However, they are not understood as a social class in the classic sense, leaving behind the relationship between social classes and health problems.

General Characteristics

The reviews were published between 2010 and 2013, and were done almost entirely by investigators from the United Kingdom. The primary studies included were developed in central and peripheral capitalist countries, predominantly European countries (**Table 1**).

Table 1
The investigators, year of publication, title, country of affiliation of the investigators, and countries of the studies included in the SR registered in the CPHG

Authors, Year	Title	Country of Affiliation of the Authors	Countries of the Studies Included
Waters et al,[15] 2011	Interventions for preventing childhood obesity	Australia, United Kingdom, Hong Kong	United States, France, Thailand, Germany, Scotland, Brazil, Ireland, Netherlands, United Kingdom, Chile, Switzerland, Mexico, Canada, Australia, New Zealand, Spain, Belgium
Dangour et al,[16] 2013	Interventions to improve water quality and supply, sanitation, and hygiene practices, and their effects on the nutritional status of children	United Kingdom, China	Pakistan, Bangladesh, Guatemala, Kenya, Ethiopia, Nigeria, Nepal, Cambodia, South Africa, Chile
Coren et al,[17] 2013	Interventions for promoting reintegration and reducing harmful behavior and lifestyles in street-connected children and young people	United Kingdom, Canada, Australia	United States, Uganda, Canada, Australia, Brazil, Egypt, Korea, Nigeria, and United Kingdom
Pega et al,[18] 2013	In-work tax credits for families and their impact on health status in adults	New Zealand, United States, United Kingdom	United States
Baker et al,[19] 2011	Community-wide interventions for increasing physical activity	Australia, United States, England	Australia, United States, Belgium, China, Norway, Netherlands, Finland, Pakistan, Canada, Denmark, Iran, France
Joyce et al,[20] 2010	Flexible working conditions and their effects on employee health and well-being	United Kingdom, Canada	Denmark, Finland, United Kingdom, Germany, Netherlands, United States, Australia
Hayes et al,[21] 2012	Collaboration between local health and government agencies for health improvement	United Kingdom	United States, Denmark, Sweden, Netherlands, Australia, Israel, Canada
Thomson et al,[22] 2013	Housing improvements for health and associated socioeconomic outcomes	United Kingdom, Canada, Australia	United Kingdom, New Zealand, Denmark, Hungary, Paraguay, Northern Ireland, Cuba, United States, Bangladesh, Germany
Turley et al,[23] 2013	Slum upgrading strategies involving physical environment and infrastructure interventions and their effects on health and socioeconomic outcomes	United Kingdom, India, United States, Germany	India, Philippines, Mexico, Argentina, Indonesia, Brazil, South Africa

Objectives of the Reviews

The primary studies of the SR present similarities in the objectives related to the effects of interventions on working and living conditions in the health of populations. Most of them comprise a set of actions arising from programs; they were not isolated actions.

Studies were conducted in the following areas:

Prevention of childhood obesity[15]

Improvements in water quality and supply, hygiene practices, and the correlation with nutritional status of children[16]

Programs for street-connected children and young people, involving inclusion and harm reduction[17]

Programs to improve incomes of workers (in-work tax credits) and the correlation with the health status of the workers[18]

Promotion of physical activity in communities[19]

The relationship between more flexible working conditions and the health and well-being of formally hired employees[20]

Collaboration between government and health agencies for the improvement of health conditions[21]

The relationship between slum upgrading, health improvements, and the socioeconomic well-being of slum dwellers in low- income and middle-income countries[22]

Housing improvements in order to enhance health and improve the socioeconomic level[23]

Theoretic Contributions of the Reviews

The examined reviews state the theoretic contributions that underlie the premises and hypotheses of the intervention, as follows:

Childhood obesity is a public health problem that is not distributed homogeneously, with high levels found in the most disadvantaged social groups. Modifiable determinants (healthy eating and active living), positive energy imbalance, and genetic, behavioral, cultural, environmental, and economic factors should be taken into account in obesity prevention intervention projects.[15]

Malnutrition is a global problem, but the highest rates are found among children in Asia and sub-Saharan Africa. Interventions should take into consideration problems involving the availability and quality of water and sanitation, the effects of these factors on the nutritional status of the population, and the associated health consequences (eg, diarrhea, environmental enteropathy, infections).[16]

Street-connected children and young people are not a homogeneous group. A logical model for primary intervention was developed with intervention components in the microenvironment, mesoenvironment, and macroenvironment, which take into account contextual factors, intermediate results, and long-term results.[17]

Social protection policies over the course of life, such as programs that encourage job retention, are recommended as effective interventions in relation to the social determinants of health. Employment and income enhance social well-being and health equity. Thus, they improve health.[18]

The logical model for interventions related to physical activity in communities indicated intermediate outcomes (knowledge of the benefits of physical activity) and long-term outcomes (reduced morbidity).[19]

Flexible working conditions are being adopted worldwide, on the assumption that they have positive effects on the productivity and health of workers. The CSDH recognizes the need for labor policies in order to improve health, including flexible working conditions. However, although employees may be interested in the possibility of achieving greater balance and control over their work, the adoption of these policies by employers may be for the purpose of increasing productivity, which can cause employees to feel insecure.[20]

Collaborations between local agencies and the health sector were proposed for implementing interventions focused on the social determinants of health. However, the SR did not find any evidence that better health resulted from this collaboration.[21]

A logical model proposes that government, private society, and civil society spheres be catalysts of policies, laws, financing, and management of slum upgrading initiatives, in order to provide enhanced quality of life in both socioeconomic and health terms.[22]

There is a strong connection between housing conditions and health. Socioeconomic factors are considered potential mediators for improving health and housing conditions. Interventions that improve housing conditions can have an impact on the dynamics established between poverty and poor health status.[23]

Methodologies Used in the New Reviews in Public Health and Old Controversies

The methodological procedures used for the SR followed Cochrane recommendations and included studies with a high level of evidence, most of them including randomized and quasirandomized clinical trials, and some accepting the inclusion of quasiexperimental studies, controlled with or without randomization, before and after trials, controlled or cross-sectional cohorts, historically controlled studies, and interrupted time series. Only 1 review was an update of a previous review.

To evaluate the levels of evidence and risk of bias of the studies, tools and checklists such as PROGRESS (Plus, place of residence, race/ethnicity/culture/language, occupation, gender/sex, religion, education, socioeconomic status, social capital, and other possible factors such as disease status or disability), Hamilton, and EPOC (The Cochrane Effective Practice and Organisation of Care), which classify evidence as low, medium, and high, were used.

The acceptance of works developed outside research designs defined as gold standard for clinical research is still in the beginning stages. Therefore, studies analyzing successful initiatives and programs in countries on the periphery of capitalism, or initiatives and programs analyzed descriptively and qualitatively from paradigmatic orientations that differ from the orientation of the natural sciences, are not included.

Most of the reviews noted that the studies had low to moderate methodological quality, likelihood of bias, heterogeneity among the interventions, and inconsistencies. Therefore, it was difficult to establish the impact of the interventions on the health of the populations under study. Applying them in practice should hence be done cautiously.

However, in some studies, it was possible to identify the impact of the evidence on health, even with a high level of bias.

Children who participated in educational, behavioral, and health promotion programs for students and parents in order to prevent obesity had a mean difference in adiposity of -0.15 kg/m^2 in relation to the control group.[15]

Interventions designed to improve the quality of water, sanitation, and hygiene resulted in a slight increase in height among children less than 5 years of age.[16]

There were favorable results from interventions geared toward street-connected children and young people, including a reduced frequency of unprotected sex among young women who participated in the intensive program; reduction, or safer use, of drugs; decreased violence; and increased contact with the family. However, the results suggest that individuals living in high-risk situations benefit from some form of structured support.[17]

Reduced tobacco use was noted among women who participated in a program to improve employment-related income.[18]

Interventions to encourage physical activity in communities did not yield consistent results in terms of improvements in health. Some studies indicated positive changes, but the results were not consistent with other studies.[19]

Interventions focusing on the needs of workers, resulting in increased control over their working conditions, are more likely to result in improvements to health and overall well-being, such as reduced blood pressure and levels of fatigue, as well as improved quality of sleep.[20]

Collaborations between local agencies for changes in the environment may produce improvements in health, although the evidence is modest. Other studies showed no reliable evidence that interventions would promote change. The studies were conducted in major capitalist countries. Those from peripheral countries did not achieve sufficient status to be part of the review. The limitations on local decisions were described, because one of the parties in the collaboration was international.[21]

Improvements in housing conditions give rise to short-term health improvements; adequate space and heating have an impact on respiratory health. The extent of health improvements is directly linked to the extent of housing improvements.[22]

Slum upgrading may reduce the incidence of diarrheal diseases and water consumption costs. The results indicated improvements related to the incidence of parasitic infections and communicable disease. There was no improvement in the income of residents or changes in unemployment levels. There was also no reliable evidence related to indicators of social participation or the support network, or perinatal maternal conditions, infant mortality, nutritional deficiencies, self-referred quality of life, education, or crime.[23]

Impact on Use

It is a challenge for researchers to evaluate the impact of the Cochrane SRs in public health. The difficulty in identifying and defining the use of Cochrane Reviews in public health is notable, as well as the need to understand how researchers use the results of these reviews.[24]

Ways to assess impact are described in the literature, and include semistructured interviews with samples of potential stakeholders on the use of the review and Internet searches by author, title, and keywords of the SR. By using these, other types of citations, such as reports, repositories, and bulletins, can be identified.[23] Annual statistics on the use of reviews, such as the number of hits and downloads, are provided by the editor of the Cochrane Library. Even so, it is difficult to measure how the results of the reviews are being used.[24]

The searches by title in 2 information sources on the Internet (Google Scholar and Web of Science) of the 9 reviews registered in the CPHG in order to verify the results and citations of these reviews are listed in **Table 2**.

Note that the publication period of the reviews (2010–2013) is likely to be a contributing factor to the number of results retrieved. To make inferences about impact using the data obtained by the search in information sources is a task that requires caution. However, it can be verified that the results of the SRs were primarily used in the preparation of articles for scientific literature in peer-reviewed journals with an emphasis on the area of public health.

Application in Research

To prevent childhood obesity, Waters and colleagues[15] claimed that it was unnecessary to continue testing short-term interventions implemented in schools for children

Table 2
Results of the Google Scholar and Web of Science searches of the titles of the 9 reviews registered in the CPHG

Categories	Results N	%
Articles from online scientific journals, non-Cochrane SRs	423	60.4
Cochrane (thematic groups, Cochrane Summaries, Wiley online, Cochrane Library reviews)	98	14.0
Books (chapters)	14	2.0
Institutions, organizations, foundations, associations (public and private)	23	3.3
Universities (theses, dissertations, documents, bulletins)	47	6.7
Web of Science	95	13.6
Total	**700**	**100**

aged 6 to 12 years with the goal of changing individual behaviors. However, the same is not the case with interventions geared toward children aged 0 to 5 years and adolescents. Improvements are needed in the following areas: (1) research and evaluation designs, (2) capturing the implementation process, (3) results in terms of measurement of equity, (4) long-term results, and (5) potential damages and costs. Research must therefore identify the effective components of an intersectorial intervention.

There is a need to evaluate long-term evidence and define the timing of interventions in childhood and the period during which interventions have the greatest impact on nutritional results.[16]

Despite the existence of relevant programs for children and young people, no vigorous evaluations with strict criteria for inclusion in the SR were identified. A limitation was noted regarding the lack of studies with a control group composed of children and young people who do not receive any type of intervention, which is the situation of most street-connected children and young people in the world. A need to conduct research in peripheral countries was noted.[17]

Studies are needed outside the United States, with a larger and more diversified range of participants. Moreover, men and other subgroups that represent important categories of the population in terms of ethnicity, income, and family type should be included in the studies.[18]

Because of the inconsistency of the results, it would be beneficial to develop new studies with different methodologies to come up with a probable result that could be applied in different populations.[19]

Future research should include study designs that explore causality and prospectively verify measurements of objective effects with clear periods of follow-up, and that use strategies for achieving results in different social groups. There is evidence that interventions involving flexible working conditions may be relevant for low-income workers and could have an impact on inequity. Future reviews should expand the analysis of the effects of interventions in more flexible working conditions, taking into consideration results such as job performance, job satisfaction, and worker morale.[20]

Despite the enthusiasm of the agencies, there are difficulties in obtaining strong evidence. Proposals for overcoming the weaknesses include (1) describing in greater detail the implementation of the programs, (2) using more robust research designs, and (3) developing integrated evaluation processes. The challenge lies in harmonizing the objectives and working methods, and monitoring and evaluation before the program is implemented, thereby protecting its fidelity and increasing its potential effectiveness.[21]

The inclusion of other types of studies was mentioned by Thomson and colleagues[22] in light of the potential of qualitative data to identify nonprespecified impacts on health questionnaires and the most immediate socioeconomic determinants of health.

New research should use reliable, objective, and comparable measurements to determine the results for health, quality of life, and socioeconomic well-being resulting from slum upgrading. The authors suggest improving research designs through uniformity of evaluation, and, for evaluative studies, to incorporate procedural and qualitative information, along with quantitative data, to determine which intervention works, and for whom.[23]

REFERENCES

1. Killoran A, Kelly MP. Evidence-based public health: effectiveness and efficiency. 2009. Oxford (United Kingdom): Oxford Scholarship Online; 2010. Available at: http://books.google.com.br/books?hl=pt-BR&lr=&id=cZegcmBkhewC&oi=fnd &pg=PR11&dq=Killoran+A,+Kelly+MP.+Evidence-based+public+health:+ effectiveness+and+efficiency.+2009&ots=-ao8I0PO1G&sig=N4AHdQerBjPIz C0MnY1I9dbBMMI#v=onepage&q=Killoran%20A%2C%20Kelly%20MP.%20 Evidence-based%20public%20health%3A%20effectiveness%20and%20efficiency. %202009&f=false. Accessed September 12, 2014.
2. Bambra C. Real world reviews: a beginner's guide to undertaking systematic reviews of public health policy interventions. J Epidemiol Community Health 2011;65:14–9.
3. Waters E, Dayle J, Jackson N, et al. Evaluating the effectiveness of public health interventions: the role and activities for the Cochrane Collaboration. J Epidemiol Community Health 2006;60:285–9.
4. World Health Organization. Commission on social determinants of health – final report. Closing the gap in a generation. The commission's overarching recommendations. p. 10. Available at: http://whqlibdoc.who.int/hq/2008/WHO_IER_ CSDH_08.1_eng.pdf. Accessed September 12, 2014.
5. Cochrane Public Health Review Group. Recommendations from the who commission on social determinants of health – Cochrane Public Health Review Group's ongoing and planned reviews of relevance. Available at: http://ph.cochrane.org/Files/CSDH %20Recommendation_PHRG%20alignment.pdf. Accessed September 12, 2014.
6. Kawachi I. Expert consultation for measurement knowledge network. Report of proceedings and recommendations. In: Commission on Social Determinants of Health – final report. Available at: http://www.who.int/social_determinants/the commission/finalreport/en/index.html. Accessed January 11, 2014.
7. Pearson A, Field J, Jordan Z. Evidence-based clinical practice in nursing and healthcare: assimilating research, experience and expertise. Oxford (United Kingdom): Blackwell; 2007. Available at: http://books.google.com.br/books? id=GKiyUfcO9H0C&printsec=frontcover&dq=inauthor:%22Alan+Pearson%22& hl=pt-BR&sa=X&ei=5AoSVOiXMreHsQT_I4C4DA&ved=0CCcQ6AEwAQ#v= onepage&q&f=false. Accessed September 12, 2014.
8. Soares CB, Campos CM, Yonekura T. Marxismo como referencial teórico-metodológico em saúde coletiva: implicações para a revisão sistemática e síntese de evidências. Rev Esc Enferm USP 2013;47:1403–9.
9. Brownson RC, Fielding JE, Maylahn CM. Evidence-based public health: a fundamental concept for public health practice. Annu Rev Public Health 2009;30: 175–201.

10. Deeks JJ, Higgins JPT, Altman DG. Analysing data and undertaking meta-analyses. In: Higgins JPT, Green S, editors. Cochrane Handbook for Systematic Reviews of Interventions version 5.0.1 (updated 2011 March). Chapter 9. The Cochrane Collaboration. p. 243–96. Available from www.cochrane-handbook. org. Accessed January 11, 2014.

11. Glasziou P, Vandenbroucke J, Chalmers I. Assessing the quality of research. BMJ 2004;328:39–41.

12. Armstrong R, Waters E, Doyle J. Reviews in health promotion and public health. In: Higgins JP, Green S, editors. Cochrane handbook for systematic reviews of interventions version 5.1.0 (updated 2011 March). Chapter 21. The Cochrane Collaboration. p. 593–606. Available at: www.cochrane-handbook.org. Accessed January 11, 2014.

13. Noyes J, Popay J, Pearson A, et al, on behalf of the Cochrane Qualitative Research Methods Group. Qualitative research and Cochrane Reviews. Chapter 20. In: Higgins JP, Green S, editors. Cochrane handbook for systematic reviews of interventions. Chichester (United Kingdom): John Wiley & Sons; 2008. p. 1–18.

14. The University of Adelaide, The Joanna Briggs Institute. Joanna Briggs Institute reviewers' manual 2014. Adelaide (South Australia): The Joanna Briggs Institute; 2014.

15. Waters E, de Silva-Sanigorski A, Burford BJ, et al. Interventions for preventing obesity in children. Cochrane Database Syst Rev 2011;(12). CD001871. Available at: http://cochrane.bireme.br/cochrane/show.php?db=reviews&mfn=960&id=CD001871&lang=pt&dblang=&lib=COC&print=yes. Accessed September 12, 2014.

16. Dangour AD, Watson L, Cumming O, et al. Interventions to improve water quality and supply, sanitation and hygiene practices, and their effects on the nutritional status of children. Cochrane Database Syst Rev 2013;(8). CD009382. Available at: http://cochrane.bireme.br/cochrane/show.php?db=reviews&mfn=5623&id=CD009382&lang=pt&dblang=&lib=COC&print=yes. Accessed September 12, 2014.

17. Coren E, Hossain R, Pardo Pardo J, et al. Interventions for promoting reintegration and reducing harmful behaviour and lifestyles in street-connected children and young people. Cochrane Database Syst Rev 2013;(2). CD009823. Available at: http://cochrane.bireme.br/cochrane/show.php?db=reviews&mfn=5791&id=CD009823&lang=pt&dblang=&lib=COC&print=yes. Accessed September 12, 2014.

18. Pega F, Carter K, Blakely T, et al. In-work tax credits for families and their impact on health status in adults. Cochrane Database Syst Rev 2013;(8). CD009963. Available at: http://cochrane.bireme.br/cochrane/show.php?db=reviews&mfn=5838&id=CD009963&lang=pt&dblang=&lib=COC&print=yes. Accessed September 12, 2014.

19. Baker PR, Francis DP, Soares J, et al. Community wide interventions for increasing physical activity. Cochrane Database Syst Rev 2011;(4). CD008366. Available at: http://cochrane.bireme.br/cochrane/show.php?db=reviews&mfn=5098&id=CD008366&lang=pt&dblang=&lib=COC&print=yes. Accessed September 12, 2014.

20. Joyce K, Pabayo R, Critchley JA, et al. Flexible working conditions and their effects on employee health and well-being. Cochrane Database Syst Rev 2010;(2). CD008009. Available at: http://cochrane.bireme.br/cochrane/show.php?db=reviews&mfn=4898&id=CD008009&lang=pt&dblang=&lib=COC&print=yes. Accessed September 12, 2014.

21. Hayes SL, Mann MK, Morgan FM, et al. Collaboration between local health and local government agencies for health improvement. Cochrane Database Syst Rev 2012;(10). CD007825. Available at: http://cochrane.bireme.br/cochrane/show.php?db=reviews&mfn=4789&id=CD007825&lang=pt&dblang=&lib=COC&print=yes. Accessed September 12, 2014.

22. Thomson H, Thomas S, Sellstrom E, et al. Housing improvements for health and associated socio-economic outcomes. Cochrane Database Syst Rev 2013;(2). CD008657. Available at: http://cochrane.bireme.br/cochrane/show.php?db=reviews&mfn=5266 &id=CD008657&lang=pt&dblang=&lib=COC&print=yes. Accessed September 12, 2014.

23. Turley R, Saith R, Bhan N, et al. Slum upgrading strategies involving physical environment and infrastructure interventions and their effects on health and socio-economic outcomes. Cochrane Database Syst Rev 2013;(1). CD010067. Available at: http://cochrane.bireme.br/cochrane/show.php?db=reviews&mfn=5864&id=CD 010067&lang=pt&dblang=&lib=COC&print=yes. Accessed September 12, 2014.

24. Armstrong R, Pettman T, Burford B, et al. Tracking and understanding the utility of Cochrane Reviews for public health decision-making. J Public Health (Oxf) 2012; 34:309–13.

Impact of Evidence and Health Policy on Nursing Practice

Bart Geurden, RN, PhD[a,b,c,d,*], Jef Adriaenssens, RN, MSc[c,d,e,f,g], Erik Franck, RN, PhD[a,b]

KEYWORDS

- Evidence-based practice • Nursing • Health policy • Microsystem
- Nurse educators

KEY POINTS

- The story of evidence-based practice in nursing is long, with many successes, contributors, leaders, scientists, and enthusiasts.
- Nurse educators have great advantages offered from a wide variety of educational resources for evidence-based practice.
- These resources offer students the opportunity to connect their emerging competencies with clinical needs for best practices in clinical and microsystem changes.

INTRODUCTION

The history of nursing reveals a pattern of recurrent issues that the profession has been required to address over time. Some of these issues included autonomy for nurses, maintenance of standards for the profession, and maintenance of control of professional nursing practice. Over time, the profession has also addressed phenomena such as nursing staff shortages, integration of new categories of health care

Disclosures: None.
[a] Department of Health Care, Karel de Grote University College, Van Schoonbekestraat 146, Antwerp 2018, Belgium; [b] Faculty of Medicine and Health Sciences, Centre for Research and Innovation in Care (CRIC), University of Antwerp, Universiteitsplein 1, Wilrijk 2610, Belgium; [c] Belgian Interuniversity Collaboration for Evidence-based Practice (BICEP), Joanna Briggs Collaboration Affiliated Centre, Kapucijnenvoer 33, blok J, bus 7001, Leuven 3000, Belgium; [d] Centre for Evidence-Based Medicine(CEBAM), Belgian Branch of the Dutch Cochrane Centre, Kapucijnenvoer 33, blok J, bus 7001, Leuven 3000, Belgium; [e] Health Psychology Unit, Institute of Psychology, Leiden University, Rapenburg 70, Leiden 2311 EZ, The Netherlands; [f] Platform Science & Practice, Vergotesquare 43, Brussel 1030, Belgium; [g] EBMPracticenet, Brussel 1030, Belgium
* Corresponding author. University of Antwerp, Faculty of Medicine and Health Sciences, Campus DE R3.32 Universiteitsplein 1, Wilrijk 2610, Belgium.
E-mail address: bart.geurden@uantwerpen.be

Nurs Clin N Am 49 (2014) 545–553
http://dx.doi.org/10.1016/j.cnur.2014.08.009
0029-6465/14/$ – see front matter © 2014 Elsevier Inc. All rights reserved.
nursing.theclinics.com

providers, and ethical dilemmas. Each decade has brought new insight into how the profession can better meet these challenges.

In recent years, one of the undeniable major developments in health care is the advent of the evidence-based practice (EBP) movement. Today, EBP is widely recognized as a key feature of modern health care. EBP and clinical practice guidelines have become increasingly known to the international health care community since the 1990s. In the early days of EBP, the translation of new knowledge into practice was the sole responsibility of the leaders of the system or teams. Currently, the expectation is that all members of the team, including nurses, must be trained in understanding what evidence is, how it can be appraised, and how it can be adapted to be used in a particular context.[1]

However, the implementation of recommended evidence-based knowledge within patient care procedures does not automatically translate into nursing practice.[2-5] Therefore, attention is now moving to the question: how to create the right conditions within the context, the team, and in the attitudes, motivation, understanding, and actions of individual health care workers to achieve changes in practice.[6-8] Incredible developments in the synthesis and use of evidence in health care over the last several years have occurred, yet the accompanying science and emerging practices that underpin evidence-based health care are often poorly understood by policymakers and health professionals. This article examines the best available evidence for nurses and critically discusses the impact of evidence and health policy on nursing education, practice, and research.

NURSES AND EVIDENCE

The most frequently used definition of evidence-based medicine from Sackett and colleagues[9] can be applied to all health care disciplines. Applied to nursing, it states, "integrating the best available research evidence with information about patient preferences, nurses' skills level, and available resources to make decisions about patient care." Such an approach to decision-making is in contrast to tradition-based decision-making or opinion-based decision-making that is based primarily on personal values and resources. Moreover, the increased emphasis on efficiency, controlling costs, and quality in health care delivery systems is rapidly changing, together with the advancement of science and technology, thereby increasing the need for reliable, up-to-date evidence about effective nursing interventions. The EBP process brought with it shifts in the research-to-practice effort, including new evidence formats (systematic reviews [SR]), new roles (knowledge brokers and transformers), new team compositions (interprofessional, frontline, mid management, and upper management), new practice cultures (self-learning teams and organizations), and new fields of science to build the "evidence on evidence-based practice."[10]

The first resource for finding high-quality SRs of the effectiveness of different types of interventions is the *Cochrane Database of Systematic Reviews* (CDSR) housed in the Cochrane Library. The library offers all health care providers, including nurses, the best quantitative evidence currently available for clinical decision-making in the form of SRs to provide the most consistent care for patients (visit: http://www.thecochranelibrary.com). The perceptions some people have that the contents of the CDSR are not relevant to nonmedical professions such as nursing are incorrect, with nearly a quarter of reviews being of some relevance to nursing care.[11] The number of SRs in the CDSR continues to increase annually, and reviews are becoming more complex (ie, with a meta-analysis). However, there is a need for more primary studies to be conducted in nursing care such as those that focus on care to produce

SRs and meta-analyses relevant to nurses. Nevertheless, there are reviews of relevance to nursing care available in the CDSR, only they might be hard to find. Enhancing the visibility of the Cochrane Library in general and the visibility of nursing-related topics within SRs will increase its use by nursing staff. The Cochrane Nursing Care Field (CNCF), officially registered with the Cochrane Collaboration on March 25, 2009, is ideally situated to facilitate this work because its primary mission is to increase the uptake of the Cochrane Library by nurses and others involved in delivering, leading, or researching nursing care. The CNCF evidence transfer program consists of the development of summaries of nursing-care-relevant *Cochrane Reviews* and their publication in "Cochrane Corner" columns of journals and Podcasts (visit http://cncf.cochrane.org/). Since 2010, more than 175 Cochrane Corner columns have been published in 25 nursing journals.

However, it is worth pointing out that the SR in the CDSR are of randomized controlled trials (RCT), and although it is possible to perform sound systematic literature reviews of other types of research (eg, qualitative research), those types of reviews are not included in the Cochrane Library. Nursing care is complex and, although reviews of this nature are useful, they are not the only type of review needed. Questions pertaining to the experience of a patient and the appropriateness of providing treatment and care are just as important in nursing care. These questions cannot be answered by RCTs and require analysis of different types of evidence that are not covered in the Cochrane database. In this regard, the approach of the Joanna Briggs Institutes (JBI) to evidence-based health care is rather unique (visit: http://joannabriggs.org). Like the Cochrane Collaboration, the JBI is an independent, international, not-for-profit research organization. It is based within the Faculty of Health Sciences at the University of Adelaide, South Australia. The number of groups collaborating with the JBI and adopting the JBI methods and methodologies is increasing, with currently 82 entities from across the globe. From this perspective, JBI is comparable with the Cochrane Collaboration. Nevertheless, in the JBI approach to evidence-based health care, it is recognized that clinical decision-making is a complex process that needs to include, but is not restricted to, evidence, context, client preference, and clinical judgment. However, it may be that the entry of EBP in the health care improvement scene is part of a major shift in paradigms: a shift that becomes apparent in the way nurses begin to think about research results, the way that nurses frame the context for improvement, and the way nurses use change to transform health care.

IMPACT ON NURSING EDUCATION

EBP, the rapid changes in health care, the shifting population needs, and the acute nursing shortages have fueled fundamental and profound changes in nursing education. In 1965, the American Nurses Association (ANA) published a position paper urging that all nursing education take place in institutions of higher education and that the minimum preparation for beginning professional nursing practice should be a baccalaureate degree education in nursing.[12,13] The first known university-based education program for nurses was founded in the 1920s in New Zealand.[14] It was not until the 1950s that such programs started to spread to North America, where the first was set up at the University of Minnesota. In the 1980s, similar processes started in Australasia. In Europe, the shift of nursing education to the universities was slower. The University of Edinburgh was the first European institution to offer a nursing degree in 1972. The new trends were readily accepted in Spain, which introduced the bachelor's degree as the minimum requirement for entry into nursing in 1989. The United

Kingdom and Ireland completed the shift to university-based education, at the diploma level, for the basic education of both nurses and midwives in 1996.[15]

In 2001, the US Institute of Medicine (IOM) published the influencing Crossing the Quality Chasm report.[16] This report prompted experts to emphasize that the preparation of health professionals was crucial to bridging the quality chasm. Later, in the IOM Health Professions Education report,[17] it was declared that current educational programs do not adequately prepare nurses, physicians, pharmacists, or other health care professionals to provide the highest quality and safest health care possible. The conclusion was that education for all health professions were in need of "a major overhaul" to prepare health professions with new skills to assume new roles.[17] In 2010, the IOM published, "The future of nursing: leading change, advancing health."[18] One conclusion of this report was that nursing curricula should include EBP. However, merely educating nurses about evidence is not enough to embed it in daily practice and in attitudes. To translate research into better outcomes, health professionals require core skills to interpret, apply, and evaluate evidence.[3,4,7,19–21]

The conclusions of the cited IOM reports require changes in the way that health professionals are educated in both academic and practice settings, to be able to focus on evidence-based quality improvement processes. Although the nature of nursing education and nursing qualifications still vary considerably across the world, most nursing faculties have developed a new and adapted competency-based curriculum integrating theory with learning from experience gained on the job. Both parts of the curriculum are of equal importance and both should become increasingly evidence-based, as research in nursing develops. The IOM urged leaders in all health disciplines to reform education in such a way that it addresses 5 core competencies essential in bridging the quality chasm: all health professionals should be educated to deliver patient-centered care as members of an interdisciplinary team emphasizing EBP, quality improvement approaches, and informatics.[17] Currently, nursing students and faculty are expected to be able to use information technology effectively and to use data and knowledge in their daily practice.[22] Moreover, a consensus is growing that, in the clinical practice, it is essential to use an information system. Besides documenting the nursing care provided, this information system should reflect the reality of the whole process of care, contributing to the research and allowing the assessment of its quality and of its continuous improvement. Professional development programs have become widely available to update skills of those professionals who are already in practice. National and international professional organizations promote and support EBP through their publications (eg, the Royal College of Nursing [RCN] http://www.rcn.org.uk/; the ANA http://www.nursingworld.org/; the International Council of Nurses http://www.icn.ch/; and many others).

EBP also demands changes in teaching itself. Although nursing education has a body of knowledge on which nurse educators base their teaching, educational strategies, and curricular designs, most of this knowledge is tacit, experiential, and based on often personal educational practice. This knowledge relates to the art of teaching in nursing and can warrant the practice of nurse educators. However, research is also necessary to demonstrate the effectiveness of teaching approaches and new educational strategies. Nurse educators need to develop the science of nursing education through qualitative and quantitative research, to add to the tacit knowledge underpinning nursing education strategies.[23] The involvement of every educator in this process will help create institutional valuing that serves to attract and retain inquisitive and reflective educators in university colleges and academic settings, while expanding evidence-based education in nursing.[24] Educators' persistence in educating the future workforce, and retooling the current workforce, with awareness, skills, and power to improve the systems of care hold promise for moving EBP toward the future.

IMPACT ON NURSING PRACTICE

When evidence-based medicine was proclaimed in 1992 in Canada, the concept of evidence-based nursing was not really new for the nursing profession. Before 1992, a range of key publications paved the way for the development of evidence-based nursing. A few examples are the "Conduct and Utilization of Research in Nursing" report[25] and the much discussed booklet, "Nursing Rituals. Research and Rational Actions."[26] In 1975, the RCN launched the slogan, "Nursing is a researched based profession."[27] Several international nursing journals were launched well before 1992 (eg, *American Journal of Nursing*, *International Journal of Nursing Studies*, *Canadian Journal of Nursing Research*, to name a few). These publications all raised awareness of the importance of nursing research and the use of research findings in practice. It caused a gradual shift of the focus of the nursing process from the process over language and nursing terminology to nursing-sensitive patient outcomes. Patient outcomes that are determined to be nursing sensitive are those that improve if there is a greater quantity or quality of nursing care (eg, pressure ulcers, falls, intravenous infiltrations, and adverse events, to name a few).[28] Some patient outcomes are more highly related to other aspects of institutional care, such as medical decisions and institutional policies (eg, frequency of primary C-sections, cardiac failure) and are therefore not considered "nursing-sensitive."[28]

Nurses have probably always known that their decisions have important implications for patient outcomes. Increasingly, however, they are being cast in the role of active decision-makers in health care by policymakers and other members of the multidisciplinary health care team.[29] In the United Kingdom, for example, the Chief Nursing Officer outlined 10 key tasks for nurses as part of the National Health Service's modernization agenda and the breaking down of artificial boundaries between medicine and nursing. Nurses are expected to access, appraise, as well as incorporate research evidence into their professional judgment and clinical decision-making.[30] However, despite the huge increase in the amount of research being generated within the nursing profession, the integration of research findings into practice remains problematic and the actual utilization of research is still sparse.[31,32] Many authors from different countries and contexts have explored barriers obstructing evidence-based nursing. They include time pressure, limited access to the literature, the absence of relevant literature, lack of confidence in the staff's ability to critically evaluate empiric research, limited interest in scientific inquiry, a work environment that does not support or value EBP, inadequate research resources, lack of evidence and limited authority or power to change practice based on research findings, and lack of professional attitudes toward the nursing profession.[8,19–21,33–36] A recent survey of the state of EBP in nurses indicated that, although nurses had positive attitudes toward EBP and wished to gain more knowledge and skills, they still faced significant barriers in using it in practice.[37] Hence, for EBP to be successfully adopted and sustained, nurses and other health care professionals recognize that it must be adopted not only by individual health care providers but also by microsystems and system leaders, as well as policymakers. Federal, state, local, and other regulatory and recognition actions (eg, the Magnet Recognition Program or Team Strategies and Tools to Enhance Performance and Patient Safety [TeamSTEPPS])[38] are necessary for EBP adoption. Another example is the Magnet Learning Communities (MLC). The MLC is an Internet-based collaborative for nurses engaged in improving patient care outcomes and excellence in nursing practice. The MLC provides an opportunity for nurses to connect and share best practices, resources, research, experiences, and strategies that have led to quality patient care, nursing excellence, and innovations in professional nursing practice (http://www.nursecredentialing.org/Magnet/Magnet-Learning).

At the start of the new millennium, there was a belief that nurses might underestimate the implications of the evidence-based movement.[39] Today, the increasing international engagement of nurses, and others associated with nursing care, offers much potential for advancing the uptake of relevant evidence into nursing practice.

IMPACT ON NURSING RESEARCH

Over time, nurse leaders have struggled to establish a discipline that is separate and unique from medicine. However, this could be accomplished only when nursing developed its own unique theory base and body of knowledge. In addition, technological advances in medicine called for concurrent advances in clinical nursing practice, which could be best developed and validated through research. Nursing research is designed to guide nursing practice and to improve the health and quality of life of nurses' patients. The quest for quality care and evidence-based practice has brought nursing research into the forefront. Nurses are vital and necessary participants in both the delivery and the development of evidence. Nurses highly influence the manner and magnitude of interventions and, because of their numbers, proximity to patients, and experience of holistic health factors, they are ideally placed to identify important clinical questions. Nevertheless, nurses' ability to participate in the research process needs to be developed more effectively—and collaboration fostered across disciplines. This process is a two-way process that also requires enthusiastic engagement from fellow health professionals.

Never before have the focus and formalization of moving evidence-into-practice been as sharp as it is seen in today's research on health care transformation efforts. However, for patients and health systems to fully benefit from evidence-practicing nurses, nurse researchers must lead a new movement to understand how to increase effectiveness, efficiency, safety, and timeliness of health care; how to improve health service delivery systems; and how to attain performance improvement. New scientific fields emerge from this movement, including translational and improvement science, implementation science, and health delivery systems science. Emancipation of the patient currently is the newest opportunity to further transform health care from a systems perspective.

SUMMARY

The story of EBP in nursing is long, with many successes, contributors, leaders, scientists, and enthusiasts. The impact on every aspect of nursing is huge and certainly not over yet. Nurse educators have great advantages offered from a wide variety of educational resources for EBP. These resources offer students the opportunity to connect their emerging competencies with clinical needs for best practices in clinical and microsystem changes. As they emerge from formal education, the employment of EBP in clinical environments will become more obvious. Clinical leaders in nursing have unprecedented opportunity to transform health care from a systems perspective, focusing on EBP for clinical effectiveness, patient engagement, and patient safety. Many national and international professional organizations for nurses promote and support EBP and life-long learning through their publications. Nurse scientists have to develop innovative programs of research in evidence-based quality improvement and implementation of EBP.

The current emphasis on evidence-based health care requires nurses to base their clinical practice to the greatest extent possible on research-based findings rather than on tradition, authority, intuition, or personal experience. Nevertheless, nursing will always remain a rich blend of art and science.

REFERENCES

1. Finotto S, Carpanoni M, Casadei Turroni E, et al. Teaching evidence-based practice: developing a curriculum model to foster evidence-based practice in undergraduate student nurses. Nurse Educ Pract 2013. http://dx.doi.org/10.1016/j.nepr.2013.03.021.
2. Burney M, Underwood J, McEvoy S, et al. Early detection and treatment of severe sepsis in the emergency department: identifying barriers to implementation of a protocol-based approach. J Emerg Nurs 2012;38(6):512–7.
3. Carrion M, Woods P, Norman I. Barriers to research utilisation among forensic mental health nurses. Int J Nurs Stud 2004;41(6):613–9.
4. Chan GK, Barnason S, Dakin CL, et al. Barriers and perceived needs for understanding and using research among emergency nurses. J Emerg Nurs 2011; 37(1):24–31.
5. Green SM, James EP. Barriers and facilitators to undertaking nutritional screening of patients: a systematic review. J Hum Nutr Diet 2013. http://dx.doi.org/10.1111/jhn.12011.
6. Estabrooks CA, Squires JE, Greta G, et al. Development and assessment of the Alberta Context Tool. BMC Health Serv Res 2009;9:234. Available at: http://www.biomedcentral.com/1472-6963/9/234.
7. Meijers JM, Janssen MA, Cummings GG, et al. Assessing the relationships between contextual factors and research utilization in nursing: systematic literature review. J Adv Nurs 2006;55(5):622–35.
8. Rycroft-Malone J. The PARIHS framework - A framework for guiding the implementation of evidence-based practice. J Nurs Care Qual 2004;19(4):297–304.
9. Sackett DL, Rosenberg WM, Gray JA, et al. Evidence based medicine: what it is and what it isn't. BMJ 1996;13:71–2.
10. Shojania KG, Grimshaw JM. Evidence-based quality improvement: the state of the science. Health Aff (Millwood) 2005;24(1):138–50.
11. Geurden B, Stern C, Piron C, et al. How relevant is the Cochrane Database of Systematic Reviews to nursing care? Int J Nurs Pract 2012;18(6):519–26.
12. Committee on Nursing Education ANA. American Nurses Association's first position on education for nursing. Am J Nurs 1965;65:106–7. http://dx.doi.org/10.2307/3419707.
13. Donley R, Flaherty MJ. Revisiting the American Nurses Association's first position on education for nurses. Online J Issues Nurs 2002;7:2.
14. Chick NP. Nursing research in New Zealand. West J Nurs Res 1987;9:317–34. http://dx.doi.org/10.1177/019394598700900304.
15. World Health Organization. Nurses and midwives for health; A WHO European strategy for nursing and midwifery education. Copenhagen (Denmark): WHO Regional Office for Europe; 2000.
16. Institute of Medicine. Crossing the quality chasm: a new health system for the 21st century. Washington, DC: Committee on Quality of Health Care in America; Institute of Medicine; National Academic Press; 2001.

17. Institute of Medicine, Greiner AC, Knebel E, editors. Health professions education: a bridge to quality. Washington, DC: National Academic Press; Institute of Medicine; 2003.
18. Institute of Medicine. The future of nursing: leading change, advancing health. Washington, DC: Institute of Medicine; National Academic Press; 2010.
19. Cooke L, Smith-Idell C, Dean G, et al. 'Research to practice': a practical program to enhance the use of evidence based practice at the unit level. Oncol Nurs Forum 2004;13:825–32.
20. Hannes K, Vandersmissen J, De Blaeser L, et al. Barriers to evidence-based nursing: a focus group study. J Adv Nurs 2007;60:162–71.
21. Mazurek Melnyk B, Fineout Overholt E, Fishbeck Feinstein N, et al. Nurses' perceived knowledge, beliefs, skills and needs regarding evidence-based practice: implications for accelerating the paradigm shift. Worldviews Evid Based Nurs 2004;3:185–91.
22. Gassert CA. Technology and informatics competencies. Nurs Clin North Am 2008;43(4):507–21. http://dx.doi.org/10.1016/j.cnur.2008.06.005, v.
23. Ferguson L, Day RA. Evidence-based nursing education: myth or reality? J Nurs Educ 2005;44(3):107–15.
24. Emerson RJ, Records K. Today's challenge, tomorrow's excellence: the practice of evidence-based education. J Nurs Educ 2008;47(8):359–70.
25. Horsley JA, Crane J, Crabtree MK, et al. Using research to improve nursing practice: a guide, CURN project. New York: Grune & Stratton; 1983.
26. Walsh M, Ford P. Nursing rituals. Research and rational actions. Oxford (United Kingdom); Waltham (MA): Butterworth-Heinemann Medical Ltd; 1989. ISBN 0750600977/0-7506-0097-7.
27. English I. Nursing as a research-based profession: 22 years after Briggs. Br J Nurs 1994;3:402–6.
28. ANA American Nurses Association. Available at: http://www.nursingworld.org/MainMenuCategories/ThePracticeofProfessionalNursing/PatientSafetyQuality/Research-Measurement/The-National-Database/Nursing-Sensitive-Indicators_1. Accessed October, 15, 2013.
29. Chief Nursing Officer. PL CNO (2002) 5: Implementing the NHS Plan—Ten key roles for nurses. London: Department of Health; 2002. Available at: http://www.dh.gov.uk/assetRoot/04/01/35/37/04013537.pdf.
30. Department of Health. Making a difference: strengthening the nursing, midwifery and health visiting contribution to health and healthcare. London: HMSO; 1999. Available at: http://www.dh.gov.uk/assetRoot/04/07/47/04/04074704.pdf.
31. Parkin C, Bullock I. Evidence-based health care: development and audit of a clinical standard for research and its impact on an NHS trust. J Clin Nurs 2005;14:418–25.
32. Rassool GH. Dissemination of nursing knowledge: the application of the model of change. J Addict Nurs 2005;16:79–82.
33. Ciliska DK, Pinelli J, DiCenso A, et al. Resources to enhance evidence-based nursing practice. AACN Clin Issues 2001;12:520–8.
34. Gennaro S, Hodnett E, Kearney M. Making evidence-based practice a reality in your institution. MCN Am J Matern Child Nurs 2001;26:236–44.
35. McCaughan D, Thompson C, Cullum N, et al. Acute care nurses' perceptions of barriers to using research information in clinical decision-making. J Adv Nurs 2002;39:46–60.
36. Windle PE. Moving beyond the barriers for evidence-based practice implementation. J Perianesth Nurs 2006;21:208–11.

37. Melnyk BM, Fineout-Overholt E, Gallagher-Ford L, et al. The state of evidence-based practice in US nurses: critical implications for nurse leaders and educators. J Nurs Adm 2012;42(9):410–7.
38. AHRQ (Agency for Healthcare Research and Quality), (2008). TeamSTEPPS national implementation project 2008. Available at: http://teamstepps.ahrq.gov/. Accessed March 2, 2014.
39. Jennings BM, Loan LA. Misconceptions among nurses about evidence-based practice. J Nurs Scholarsh 2001;33:121–7.

Translating Evidence into Policy and Practice

Craig Lockwood, RN, BN, GDipClinN, MNSc, PhD[a],*, Edoardo Aromataris, BSc, PhD[b],
Zachary Munn, BMedRad(NucMed), GDHSc, PhD[a]

KEYWORDS

- Translation science • Knowledge to action • Joanna Briggs Institute
- Implementation science • Evidence-based practice

KEY POINTS

- Good quality evidence from systematic reviews forms the basis for translation of evidence in to practice.
- Reliance on robust systems for transfer of knowledge facilitates sustainable delivery of evidence to the point of care.
- Practice change is as much about behavioral change as it is about the use of technology.
- An appropriate theoretic framework recognizes that evidence should respond to global needs, be based on rigorous systematic reviews, and focus on transfer of evidence appropriate to local needs.
- Clinicians need appropriate preparation in leadership and training in skills and knowledge for implementation.
- Organizations seeking to improve their evidence-based culture should seek to establish a cohort of like-minded practitioners able to advance translation of evidence into practice by providing appropriate training and support.

INTRODUCTION

Quality improvement (QI) in health care has a rich history of adapting what works from other fields and applying it. The airline industry and manufacturing are just 2 sources of models, methods, and ideas that have informed QI in health care. However, the evidence of effectiveness of our QI processes remains characterized by uncertainty and large gaps in time between what we know to be best practice and implementation.[1]

Disclosures: None.
[a] Faculty of Health Sciences, The Joanna Briggs Institute, Implementation Science, School of Translational Health Science, The University of Adelaide, North Terrace, Adelaide, South Australia 5005, Australia; [b] Faculty of Health Sciences, The Joanna Briggs Institute, School of Translational Health Science, The University of Adelaide, North Terrace, Adelaide, South Australia 5005, Australia
* Corresponding author.
E-mail address: craig.lockwood@adelaide.edu.au

Nurs Clin N Am 49 (2014) 555–566
http://dx.doi.org/10.1016/j.cnur.2014.08.010
0029-6465/14/$ – see front matter © 2014 Elsevier Inc. All rights reserved.

Given that these issues seem to be resistant to concerted efforts to address QI and patient safety, it may be useful to examine how frameworks from other fields can be adapted to fit translational practices for evidence-based health care. Six Sigma is one such framework.

Six Sigma is the Japanese manufacturing framework that revolutionized that country's industry, wealth, and reputation and accelerated Japan to second place, only behind the United States, as the world's most powerful economy.[2] Despite initially being largely the domain of manufacturing and technology, the impact of Six Sigma has been felt around the world; its methods have been adopted and adapted, and its influence is now felt across many sectors. This impact of Six Sigma is not just driven by management and company chief executives; Six Sigma only works when there is high uptake of the methods and values across an entire organization. Six Sigma spans manufacturing, information technology, health, and education, to name just a few fields. Although not without its critics, the awarding of Six Sigma status has long been recognized as a gold standard achievement.

But not all that glitters is gold, nor is Six Sigma status the only benchmark for better practice in industry. Enter the city of Mumbai's food distribution system, where every day around 4000 Dabbawallahs' pick up cooked lunches from suburban homes, hand delivering over 200,000 home-cooked lunches across the city. Estimates indicate that for every 6 million *tiffins* (lunch boxes) delivered and returned, there is 1 error, a reliability rate of greater than 99.9% for quality (available from http://mumbaidabbawala.in/about-us/) and a figure that industry giants like GE, 3M, and Motorola who once aspired to Six Sigma status can only aspire to, but also one that informs questions about the basis of our approach to policy and practice for care delivery in the health professions.

Certainly, health care is characterized by extensive, complex sectors designed to address the health needs of countries, states, and counties right down to rural and remote communities and specific, vulnerable groups in society. Health care services are highly regulated; they consist of integrated networks of staff across professions and are exposed to high costs for new equipment, constantly updated care practices, and health professionals who are subject to regular reviews.

The frameworks we adopt and implement for the transfer or translation of evidence into policy and practice can end up looking like the requirements of a manufacturing giant, or a Fortune 500 company, yet lack the outcomes of a group of highly dedicated and enthusiastic Dabbawallah's.

Not that this implies we are doing something wrong, but it does raise some points to consider. The lunch delivery system grew out of a practical need, rather than being crafted to create a perceived market. The program is structured yet flexible with immense capacity for growth and despite its size it remains people-centric. A key factor in its success seems to be its reliance on the use of the Mumbai rail system as its delivery framework. Why is this? The Mumbai rail system is reliable, efficient, and is far reaching. In health care, a framework is required that equates to the Mumbai rail system that has the reliability and capacity to deliver evidence, tools, systems, and resources across the health industry, responsively, with immense capacity for growth, to networks, groups, and individuals. Having the right framework in place is arguably a fundamental for effective evidence-informed health care policy and practice.

THE TRANSLATIONAL HEALTH CYCLE

The Joanna Briggs Institute (JBI) characterizes translation science as a process arising from a need, specifically, the need to move research findings in to policy and practice.[3] Pearson and colleagues[3] go on to indicate that although increasing volumes of literature are published on translation science, much of it represents white noise and may actually confound the best attempts to achieve evidence-informed policy and practice. The core elements of translation science begins with a global health need; primary research generates evidence related to meeting health care needs and this research can be synthesized through systematic reviews and then translated into summative papers such as guidelines. These guidelines then facilitate dissemination of research evidence, the utilization of research evidence, and the evaluation of impact on outcomes (**Fig. 1**). However, the language to describe these elements varies enormously in the published literature, as does the number of steps in the translational cycle, and modes by which knowledge (evidence) is transferred to knowledge users. Much of this variation is captured, evaluated, and clearly communicated in the work of Pearson and colleagues[3] (2011) and Graham and colleagues[4] (2006), and is not be revisited herein.

As Pearson and colleagues[3] describe, translation of evidence into practice is a cyclical process. The process begins with identifying clinically relevant questions or health care needs, followed by identifying and reviewing all available evidence for quality and applicability to specific populations and health policy or practice. This requires the transparent and rigorous process found in systematic review methodology, which is the most reliable basis for identifying evidence for translation in to practice. A systematic review that attempts to include all international research, both published

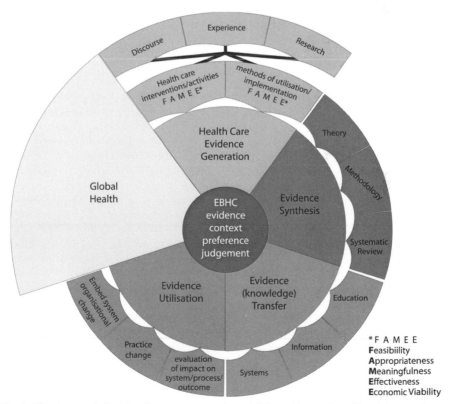

Fig. 1. The Joanna Briggs Institute conceptual model for evidence-based health care. (*Courtesy of* the Joanna Briggs Institute, The University of Adelaide, South Australia, Australia; with permission.)

and unpublished (gray) is at lower risk of publication bias, and is therefore better placed than single studies to present reliable measures of precision and magnitude for evidence of effects and better able to present a robust understanding of other forms of evidence, such as economic or qualitative findings. Despite the advantages of systematic reviews, without an appropriate model for translation, the evidence they present to the decision makers for evidence-informed health care may not gain traction in health care policy or practice.

The JBI model links continuous developments in systematic review methodology with the needs of health professionals for rigorous systems and resources at the point of care to facilitate access and enable active uptake of evidence. Systematic review findings are rapidly translated into guidelines, evidence summaries, consumer (patient) information, educational programs and activities, resources for QI, indicators for collection of key performance metrics indicators, and indicators for JBI evidence-based clinical audits. This translational cycle can be conceptualized as the delivery system, arising from a pragmatic need to transfer high quality evidence about specific outcomes across complex environments. The following example of moving from published systematic review to clinical practice guideline to implementation and evaluation of outcomes illustrates how a robust evidence base can be transferred in to practice based on the JBI model for evidence-based health care. The second half of this paper presents the methodology and theory for the differing components of the case study, that is, the evidence and theory for systematic reviews, the transfer of systematic review findings into accessible guidance, and the impact of having point-of-care resources available to support clinicians who are appropriately trained in leadership and evidence-based practice.

Case Study: Pediatric Fever

Pediatric fever is a common cause of parental anxiety that leads to increased health provider visits for little benefit to the patient, particularly in the absence of symptoms that indicate a potentially serious diagnosis.[5] Evidence suggests fever is the reason for up to 30% of pediatric consultations, often owing to a lack of clear parental understanding of treatment options, and that presentation to a health setting with fever may result in excessive administration of antipyretics. Compounding the level of burden on families and health systems is the lack of clarity around what temperature indicates the presence or absence of fever.

Families tend to move quickly to pharmacotherapy, without being clear on the longer term risks from medication use.[5] The long-term effects of childhood exposure to acetaminophen or ibuprofen are unclear, but seem to include increased risk of asthma and allergies.[5] The problem is global; families lack access to evidence about effective nonpharmacologic strategies to manage fever in otherwise healthy children.

A JBI systematic review published in 2012 sought to establish the effectiveness of nonpharmacologic therapies for the treatment of febrile episodes in children aged from 3 months to 12 years.[5] The review used a comprehensive search of the international literature to identify randomized controlled trials published between 2001 and 2012 in English, Spanish, Portuguese, Mandarin, or Italian. A total of 12 randomized controlled trials were included after detailed screening and critical appraisal. The review aimed to report on the effect on fever, changes in comfort, differences in parental anxiety, and changes in use of health services. The interventions reported in the included studies were the use of direct external cooling measures, with some studies also including sponging or the removal of layers of clothing. No studies explicitly investigated hydration, rest, or use of fans or other cooling devices, and only 2 of the outcomes included in the a priori protocol were reported in the studies (effect on fever and patient comfort).[5]

Identified studies that met the inclusion criteria were subject to critical appraisal by 2 independent reviewers who did not confer during the appraisal process to ensure independent evaluation of the quality (internal validity) of studies. Data related to individual study characteristics, methods, and samples were then extracted, along with numeric data related to the specific outcomes of interest to the review. Data were extracted using standardized templates embedded in the JBI-SUMARI software.[6] Use of standardized instruments for critical appraisal and data extraction promotes consistency between reviewers, and more reliable decisions regarding both the quality of studies being included, and the reliability and accuracy of the data being extracted for analysis.[6]

The review reported a detailed analysis of study quality, methods, participant characteristics, types of interventions, how the interventions were administered, how outcomes were measured, and duration of follow-up. The specific comparisons addressed in the review were:

- Sponging compared with antipyretic only (paracetamol; 7 studies)
- Sponging compared with antipyretic plus sponging (6 studies)
- Antipyretic compared with antipyretic plus sponging (9 studies).

Owing to differences in how the interventions were administered, the review results were presented as a narrative summary rather than a pooled statistical analysis (meta-analysis). Presentation of results as a narrative summary creates challenges in interpreting and disseminating the findings, because the results must be presented as a comprehensive whole, without combining individual study results. Lockwood and White[7] describe a number of techniques and strategies for overcoming challenges in the presentation of narrative data.

The results of the review showed that antipyretics were more effective than sponging for temperature reduction within the first 60 minutes, although after 1 hour only 3 studies found a significant difference favoring pharmacotherapy alone. Five studies showed that the combination of pharmacotherapy plus sponging was more effective than sponging alone with an additional temperature decrease ranging from 0.4°C to 0.6°C. However, the duration of effect from sponging was short, with no long-term impact on temperature noted.[5] Other key findings from the review were that that when antipyretic therapy was administered with sponging, there was no clear clinical benefit compared with antipyretic alone at 2 hours post therapy. Considering the 'child's comfort,' analysis of this outcome showed sponging increased discomfort in studies, and no studies found sponging increased comfort. The final outcome of interest reported in the review was parental acceptability, and antipyretics scored the highest level of parental acceptance compared with any other intervention.[5]

Making sense of a research result where for 1 outcome, 3 studies show a favorable result, and 2 others show no difference is a complex and nuanced process. Presenting the results of systematic reviews as a series of variable findings creates challenges for those reading, seeking to interpret the results and attempting to establish the relevance to policy or practice.[7] Although reviews are considered the optimal basis for evidence-informed policy or practice, many find that the presentation confounds their ability to understand and interpret of the results in a meaningful way.[7] Therefore, a JBI systematic review also provides recommendations that are worded to reflect the information needs of practitioners and avoid the 'jargonistic' language of science that has been shown to decrease use of research findings. However, presenting recommendations provides a clinically relevant medium. An example recommendation from this review:

The routine use of sponging to reduce fever is not supported (Level II). However, providing the parent with the opportunity to bath a child who enjoys it, and who shows no signs of discomfort, may alleviate parental anxiety. It may also make the child feel more comfortable (Level III).

A JBI Clinical Fellow reports on an implementation project that sought to 'promote evidence based best practice management of febrile illness in children less than 5 years at the Limbe Health Center in Malawi and thereby improve health of children and their caregivers.'[8(p258)] Although fever in otherwise healthy children can lead to treatments that cause discomfort, in environments where there is a high burden of disease, morbidity and mortality associated with childhood fevers, untreated fever can significantly worsen health outcomes.[8]

The project used a 3-phase clinical audit approach beginning with establishing a multidisciplinary team to engage in the project and participate in baseline audit data collection. A detailed description of the audit methods can be read in the JBI Database of Systematic Reviews and Implementation Reports.[8]

A total of 5 systematic reviews informed the development of audit criteria in this project, and current practice was then measured at project baseline against the following standards:

1. A full assessment of the child is carried out to predict risk of serious illness
2. Antipyretics are administered as clinically indicated
3. During triage, the temperature of the child is taken to assess for presence of fever
4. Parents/carers are given information on fever management before discharge from the outpatient department.

The Practical Application of Clinical Evidence System (PACES, an online clinical audit software program) was utilized to collect and analyze data. PACES generates real-time results as raw data are entered into the audit system. The emerging compliance data indicated 45% adherence to best practice for criteria 1 and 3 and, 0% for criteria 2 and 4 during the baseline audit. These data were presented to facility staff in the context of exploring and seeking to identify strategies that would assist with evidence-based practice change in the management of children with fever. Although audit programs commonly establish a measurement of compliance against a standard, PACES specifically includes standards derived from high-quality, systematic reviews to ensure each criteria represents best practice.[9]

In this case study, the barriers identified through group analysis were:

- Lack of knowledge specific to fever assessment and diagnosis by triage staff
- Availability of antipyretics and thermometers
- Lack of standardized assessment tools
- Lack of standardized guidance for when to implement different interventions.

For each barrier, a series of strategies was identified and implemented, the GRiP process (Getting Research into Practice; a guided method of situational analysis built into PACES) was also used to identify and respond to resource implications for each strategy. The implementation phase continued for 2 months before a follow-up clinical audit using the same criteria, methods, and sample size was conducted. Compliance data showed that practice was substantially more concordant with best practice, with 90% adherence to best practice for criteria 1 and 100% compliance for criteria 2, 3, and 4. **Fig. 2** shows the degree of change in practice achieved through this translation science project.

The report concludes that the greatest increase in compliance was in the provision of antipyretics as clinically indicated and according to guidelines on antipyretics. Specific interventions found to be beneficial were 1-to-1 teaching sessions on clinical assessment with clinicians on duty, and provision of tools to aid assessment. Contextual factors such as high patient/staff ratios and lack of resources, in addition to clinician behavior, were found to work against best practice implementation. These highlight that context, behaviors, and beliefs have as significant a role in translation science as evidence itself does.[8]

Lessons Learned from the Case Study: Evidence Synthesis

Starting with high-quality evidence reduces the impact of barriers to practice change that may be based on resistance to or uncertainty about the quality of evidence. Systematic reviews have become recognized as the internationally accepted gold standard for generating evidence to inform policy or practice change.[3] High-quality reviews (comparative effectiveness reviews included) are recognized as scientific research that use existing literature (published and unpublished) as the data source. Systematic reviewers develop an a priori protocol to guide the conduct of their review. This, along with other features of the systematic review, contribute to their scientific validity and hence their position as level 1 evidence in evidence hierarchies around the world.[10] It is worth noting that it is not only quantitative research that can be synthesized in systematic reviews to inform policy and practice. Hannes and Lockwood[11] have previously demonstrated meta-aggregation has a high level of goodness of fit with the policy and practice needs of the health sciences as a methodology for qualitative systematic reviews. Replicating the pragmatic analytical assumptions of meta-analysis by avoiding overt user interpretation, meta-aggregation produces review findings that are intended to be used to inform policy and practice rather than generate theories for testing.[11] Similarly, in relation to evidence-informed health care, models for knowledge translation that have a focus on outcomes are able to be built on and expanded, rather than recreate frameworks for implementation of best practice. This allows users to focus on taking the knowledge they need, and selecting resources to facilitate its implementation to improve practice and patient outcomes. This focus on outcomes is at the center of an effective translational model.[4,12]

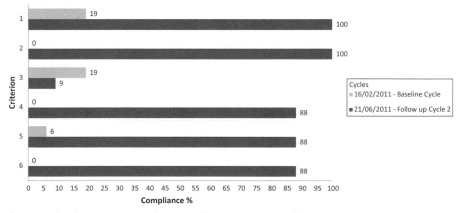

Fig. 2. Preimplementation and postimplementation compliance reports.

The role of systematic reviews as the optimal basis of and a key element in the translation of knowledge for evidence-informed health care is illustrated in the JBI conceptual model.[3] It is from high-quality reviews that evidence is identified and translated into accessible forms and formats, suited to the transfer of knowledge into tools and resources suited to point-of-care applications. Without an objectively developed, comprehensive body of knowledge as the basis for decision making, recommendations for practice increase in reliance on individual expertise of the health professional, leading to variability in practice.[13]

JBI systematic reviews use internationally accepted and recognized methodology and methods for each step in the process.[6] However, given the organizational mandate is to promote evidence-based health care, JBI reviews go beyond presenting findings. Each JBI review also includes recommendations for policy and practice, where the recommendations are graded based on the strength and rigor of the underlying evidence.[6]

Lessons Learned from the Case Study: Evidence Transfer

The availability of systematic review findings to end-users has been found to be low.[14] Guideline developers in particular seek to transfer the evidence into forms and formats that are more suited to the particular information needs of clinicians. One approach to transforming systematic review findings into accessible evidence for practice is the highly successful short form 'Best Practice' series.[15] These 4-page guidelines present the key contextual knowledge as well as recommendations (with their grading based on the strength of the evidence) and include an algorithm related to the decision points in transferring the knowledge to practice. Written in nonstatistical language with the topic and recommendations clearly identified on the front page, these sheets have been found to increase accessibility of evidence at the point of care.

The series is available electronically for access from any type of mobile or desktop device; each issue includes a background to convey the context for the topic, a summary of the objectives and methods reported in a systematic review, and detailed descriptions of the interventions and inclusion criteria. Keeping to a maximum of 4 pages and including an algorithm facilitates understanding and moves beyond reporting findings to presenting detailed recommendations further adds to the practical utility.

The translation of evidence from systematic reviews into accessible point-of-care knowledge through clinical practice guidelines is an established mechanism.[16] However, evidence translation is also known to be ineffective unless specific strategies are put in place to ensure knowledge is not just made available (disseminated), but also facilitate its uptake and use in practice. Translating knowledge into action (getting research into practice) requires facilitated uptake by practitioners.[16] Programmatic approaches facilitate a sustainable model for translating evidence in to practice.[16] Combining facilitation with education programs leads to the development of cohorts of clinicians with a common base of knowledge, skills, and resources to translate evidence into practice. From this approach it is often the clinician who is left out of the equation, or more precisely, it is the supportive preparation and equipping of clinicians with targeted knowledge and skills for evidence-based practice that remains unaddressed.

Undergraduate programs may provide good introductory level exposure to translation science.[17] However, exposure in undergrad programs has not been linked to sustainable impact on practice or patient outcomes.[17–19] Postgraduate programs sometimes include components that address aspects of translation science, and a few programs claim to be based entirely on translation science; however, models of education at the undergraduate and postgraduate levels both miss a cultural dynamic that is of immense benefit to an organization seeking to become an evidence-based provider of health care services.[20,21]

Organizational culture is resistant to change. Therefore, increasing the number of undergraduates or postgraduates with knowledge of translation science per university is not the same as a hospital or health care facility strategically investing in preparing a cohort of its own staff who have been equipped with the knowledge, skills, and resources to identify local needs, access the relevant evidence, and undertake multidisciplinary implementation projects that respond to local need and priorities and fit the local cultural context.

Often, health professionals end up in leadership roles feeling underprepared and facing intimidating expectations that are largely based on their clinical skills.[9,20,21] Finding the appropriate fit between academically prepared staff and organization-specific needs and priorities in practice can be a delicate balance. The solution is not always the most high tech or headline grabbing. Nor do you need to go to Mumbai to analyze transfer systems; however, appreciating that local solutions provide goodness of fit with a local context is a lesson that should not be missed. The JBI evidence-based clinical fellowship program is designed to address this gap. The program focuses on leadership skills, cultural contexts for understanding self and others, and practical techniques to create or build a culture of engagement with evidence.

Lessons Learned from the Case Study: Evidence Utilization

The evidence-based clinical fellowship program is a 6-month workplace program that includes two 5-day intensive residencies in JBI focusing on training in evidence-based practice, developing a proposal for an implementation project, and undertaking leadership training. Topics are set by each candidate in conjunction with their senior facility leadership, ensuring the strategic relevance of the topic. The fellow then helps to build a local team of health professionals grounded in applied translation science knowledge; the program models scientific strength paired with pragmatic locally derived clinical solutions to implement best practice and sustain changes over time. Audit and feedback has been shown to facilitate important changes in health care practice, therefore basing the fellowship program structure on clinical auditing with evidence-based audit criteria for compliance measurement has been validated as a mechanism for knowledge transfer.[22]

Fellowship projects use the JBI PACES, the Practical Application of Clinical Evidence System.[23] JBI PACES is an online tool for health professionals and/or researchers conducting clinical audits within one or across multiple health care settings. PACES has been designed to facilitate audits being used to promote evidence-informed health practice and includes a GRiP framework that is used to help to identify barriers to best practice and strategies to overcome them. PACES is an 'always online' system for audit and implementation where there is an organizational commitment to best practice standards as the basis of health care.

The workplace component of the program consists of a baseline clinical audit that measures current practice against best practice recommendations that have been published in systematic reviews and transferred into best practice guidance. The delivery of improvements to practice that these Fellows are able to achieve, simply by having access to the best information and a simple tool to assist them to assess and change their practice at the point of care, is best conveyed through a case study.

Compliance measures provide an indication of current organizational or unit level performance; however, practice change—the translation of evidence in to practice—requires clinicians with the knowledge, skills, and leadership to confidently lead multidisciplinary teams in the evaluation of specific barriers to better practice and the identification of strategies and resources to facilitate practice change.

Although more complex systems exist, the combination of Clinical Fellowship Training Program with regular, real-time data reporting provides clinicians with the evidence to support practice change.

However, practice change is a nuanced process, as much behavioral as it is objective science, with many local contextual variations impacting the success of strategies. As with knowledge to action models, an environmental scan or situational analysis may assist in establishing consensus about priorities for practice change and the specific strategies that might be adopted to facilitate any changes to practice.[24] The JBI-PACES software includes the module GRiP, which is a guided situational analysis module that looks at barriers to compliance, frames these in the context of barrier specific strategies, and resource identification.

DISCUSSION

A number of studies have started linking behavioral science to translation. Theoretic domains of belief and their links to behavior offer nuanced observations that can inform our understandings of how to get evidence in to practice.[3,4,22,25]

The realization that behavioral factors, beliefs, and context have a significant impact on the success of knowledge translation brings us back to the Mumbai, lunch delivering, 'Dabbawallahs.' A tendency to favor complex systems is no guarantee of success; rather, building an ethos that values best practice and building of cohorts of practitioners who are skilled and knowledgeable in translation science practices able to situate contextual factors, beliefs, and behaviors within a framework (such as the JBI model) is more likely to achieve successful translation.

The JBI systematic review program provides a robust framework for synthesis science on which to base the development of rigorous evidence for practice. Translation of evidence into policy and practice should start with this assumption that high-quality evidence is needed to form the basis for transfer of knowledge. Appropriate guidelines facilitate the dissemination of knowledge, as do online and other resources; however, moving knowledge into practice requires time and energy regardless of the nature and quality of the evidence. Maximizing the benefits is achieved through strategic use of existing, robust systems that have built-in reliability and capacity. However, knowledge translation is not just about systems; it is primarily about people, recognizing their capacity and expanding their skill sets or toolbox for the transfer of knowledge to action. The ability to influence and manage change is a taught or learned behavior.[9] The clinical fellowship program provides the skills and knowledge to work colleagues, patients, and systems to motivate, persuade, challenge, and stimulate others for a shared, practical approach to translating evidence in to practice.

This program has a persistent positive impact on policy and practice outcomes across the domains of care, including long-term care, acute care, and rural and remote settings, as well as specialist fields and scopes of practice. This compelling body of evidence relates to projects where the framework is an evidence-based model combined with teaching in clinical leadership as well as the skills and knowledge for translation of evidence in to practice.

REFERENCES

1. Sunol R, Wagner C, Arah OA, et al. Evidence-based organization and patient safety strategies in European hospitals. Int J Qual Health Care 2014;26:47–55 Pubmed Central PMCID: 24578501.
2. Zugelder TJ. Lean six sigma literature: a review and agenda for future research [Conventional]. Columbus: The Ohio State University; 2012.

3. Pearson A, Weeks S, Stern C. Translation science and the JBI model of evidence-based healthcare. In: Pearson A, editor. Philadelphia: Lippincott Williams & Wilkins; 2011. p. 67.
4. Graham ID, Logan J, Harrison M, et al. Lost in translation: time for a map? J Contin Educ Health Prof 2006;26:13–24.
5. Watts R, Robertson J. Non-pharmacological management of fever in otherwise healthy children. JBI Library of Systematic Reviews 2012;10(28):1634–87.
6. The Joanna Briggs Institute. Reviewers manual. In: The Joanna Briggs Institute, editor. Adelaide (Australia): Solito Fine Colour; 2014. p. 196.
7. Lockwood C, White SL. Synthesizing descriptive evidence. In: Pearson A, editor. Synthesis Science in Healthcare Series: Book 10. Sydney (Australia): Lippincott Williams and Wilkins; 2012. p. 57.
8. Chibwana AI, Gomersall JS. Management of febrile illness in children less than 5 years of age at Libme Health Centre, Blantyre district in Malawi: a best practice implementation project. JBI Database of Systematic Reviews and Implementation Reports 2013;11(12):256–72.
9. The Joanna Briggs Institute. The Joanna Briggs Institute fellows reports. Adelaide (Australia): The Joanna Briggs Institute; 2011. p. 295.
10. Lockwood C. Critiquing the contested nature of aggregation in qualitative evidence synthesis: an examination of dominant views on interpretivism [Conventional]. Adelaide (Australia): University of Adelaide; 2011.
11. Hannes K, Lockwood C. Pragmatism as the philosophical foundation for the Joanna Briggs meta-aggregative approach to qualitative evidence synthesis. J Adv Nurs 2011;67(7):1632–42.
12. Pentland D, Forsyth K, Maciver D, et al. Key characteristics of knowledge transfer and exchange in healthcare: integrative literature review. J Adv Nurs 2011;76(6): 1365–2648.
13. McCaughey D, Bruning NS. Rationality versus reality: the challenges of evidence-based decision making. Implement Sci 2010;5:39.
14. Pakenham-Walsh N, Priestley C. Towards equity in global health knowledge. QJM 2002;95(7):469–73.
15. The Joanna Briggs Institute. Children's experiences of postoperative pain management. The Joanna Briggs Institute Database of Best Practice Information Sheets and Technical Reports 2013;17(7):4.
16. Rotter T, Kinsman L, James EL, et al. Clinical pathways: effects on professional practice, patient outcomes, length of stay and hospital costs. Cochrane Database Syst Rev 2010;(3):CD006632.
17. Robinson BK, Dearmon V. Evidence-based nursing education: effective use of instructional design and simulation learning environments to enhance knowledge transfer in undergraduate nursing students. J Prof Nurs 2013;29(4):203–9.
18. Forsetlund L, Bjørndal A, Rashidian A, et al. Continuing education meetings and workshops: effects on professional practice and health care outcomes. Cochrane Database Syst Rev 2009;(2):CD003030.
19. Flodgren G, Rojas-Reyes MX, Cole N, et al. Effectiveness of organisational infrastructures to promote evidence-based nursing practice. Cochrane Database Syst Rev 2012;(2):CD002212.
20. Coomarasamy A, Khan KS. What is the evidence that postgraduate teaching in evidence based medicine changes anything? A systematic review. BMJ 2004;329:5.
21. Coomarasamy A, Taylor R, Khan KS. A systematic review of postgraduate teaching in evidence-based medicine and critical appraisal. Med Teach 2003;25(1): 77–81.

22. Ivers N, Jamtvedt G, Flottorp S, et al. Audit and feedback: effects on professional practice and healthcare outcomes. Cochrane Database Syst Rev 2012;(6):CD000259.
23. Munn Z, Kavanagh S, Woods F, et al. The development of an evidence-based resource for burns care. Burns 2013;39(4):577–82.
24. Graham ID. Knowledge synthesis and the Canadian Institutes of Health Research. Syst Rev 2012;1:6.
25. Francis JJ, O'Connor D, Curran J. Theories of behavior change synthesised into a set of theoretical groupings: introducing a thematic series of the theoretical domains framework. Implement Sci 2012;7:9.

Index

Note: Page numbers of article titles are in **boldface** type.

C

Campbell Collaboration, 457, 464
Cochrane Collaboration, 456, 463–464
Cumulative Index to Nursing and Allied Health Literature (CINAHL), 478–481

D

Delirium, prevention in postoperative hip fracture patients, 516–520

E

Education, impact of evidence and health policy on nursing, 547–549
Evidence synthesis, role in evidence-based health care, **453–460**
    Campbell Collaboration, 457
    emergence in the US and internationally, 454–457
    systematic review, 457–459
Evidence-based health care, 453–566
  and health policy, impact of, **545–553**
    on nursing education, 547–549
    on nursing practice, 547–549
    on nursing research, 550
  developing a robust evidence base for nursing, **475–484**
    definition and implications of, 475–477
    trends in publication of systematic reviews relevant to nursing, 477–483
  evidence synthesis and its role in, **453–460**
    Campbell Collaboration, 457
    emergence in the US and internationally, 454–457
    systematic review, 457–459
  for rehabilitation, **507–524**
  in mental health, **525–531**
  in pediatrics, **493–506**
  in perioperative care, **485–492**
  in public health, **533–544**
  systematic review of evidence, **461–473**
    definition, 461
    difference from other reviews, 461–462
    steps in, 464–472
    types of, 463
    uses of, 462–463
    where to find reviews, 463–464
  translating evidence into policy and practice, **555–566**
    case study, 558–561

Nurs Clin N Am 49 (2014) 567–571
http://dx.doi.org/10.1016/S0029-6465(14)00096-6
0029-6465/14/$ – see front matter © 2014 Elsevier Inc. All rights reserved.

nursing.theclinics.com

Evidence-based (*continued*)
    evidence synthesis, 561–562
    evidence transfer, 562–563
    evidence utilization, 563–564
  translational health cycle, 556–558

G

GRADE system, for evaluating quality of evidence, 472

H

Health policy, impact of evidence and, **545–553**
  nurses and evidence, 546–547
  on nursing education, 547–549
  on nursing practice, 547–549
  on nursing research, 550
Hip fractures, prevention of postoperative delirium after, 516–520

I

Implementation science, translating evidence into policy and practice, **555–566**
  case study, 558–561
    evidence synthesis, 561–562
    evidence transfer, 562–563
    evidence utilization, 563–564
  translational health cycle, 556–558
International nursing, emergence of evidence-based care in, 454–457
Intraoperative care, evidence in, 490

J

Joanna Briggs Institute (JBI), 456–457, 464
  bibliographic trends in nursing from library at, 481–482
  translational health cycle model from, 481–482

L

Literature review, vs systematic review, 461–462

M

Mental health, systematic review in, **525–531**
  emerging topics for, 530
  for practitioners in, 527–529
  gaps in, 529–530
  process of, 526–527
  sample of, 529

N

Nurses, evidence and, 546–547
Nursing, impact of evidence and health policy, **545–553**
 nurses and evidence, 546–547
 on nursing education, 547–549
 on nursing practice, 547–549
 on nursing research, 550
 practice. *See* Practice, nursing.

P

Pediatrics, evidence-based health care in, **493–506**
 case study, 499–504
  critical appraisal of studies reviewed, 502–503
  detailing strategy to select all relevant literature, 501–502
  developing a rigorous protocol, 500
  establishing criteria for selection of literature, 501
  extracting data from primary research, 503
  generating a meta-analysis, 503–504
  stating the review questions hypothesis, 500
 importance of quality in reporting and publishing systematic reviews,
  494–499
Perioperative care, evidence in, **485–492**
 systematic reviews in, 487–480
  case study, 491
  intraoperative care, 490
  postoperative care, 490
  preoperative care, 487
Policy. *See also* Health policy.
 translating evidence into practice and, **555–566**
  case study, 558–561
   evidence synthesis, 561–562
   evidence transfer, 562–563
   evidence utilization, 563–564
  translational health cycle, 556–558
Postoperative care, evidence in, 490
Practice, nursing, impact of evidence and health policy on, 547–550
 systematic reviews in, in pediatrics, **493–506**
  in perioperative care, **485–492**
 translating evidence into policy and, **555–566**
  case study, 558–561
   evidence synthesis, 561–562
   evidence transfer, 562–563
   evidence utilization, 563–564
  translational health cycle, 556–558
 trends in publication of systematic reviews relevant to, 477–483
Preferred Reporting Items for Systematic Reviews and Meta-analysis (PRISMA),
 462, 483
Preoperative care, evidence in, 487
Public health, evidence in, **533–544**
 case examples of systematic reviews in, 536–542

Public (*continued*)
   application in research, 540–542
   general characteristics, 536
   impact on use, 540
   methodologies and old controversies in, 540
   objectives of the reviews, 538
   theoretic contributions of, 538–539
 controversies in methodologies for synthesis of, 534–535
 recommendations for systematic reviews in, 535–536

Q

Quality, of evidence, in a systematic review, 468

R

Rehabilitation, finding and using best evidence for, acute delirium and
   systematic reviews, 516–520
      case study using systematic reviews in hip fracture care, 514–516, 520–522
      systematic reviews and clinical guidelines, 514
      where to find systematic reviews, 508–514
Research, impact of evidence and health policy on nursing, 550
Review, systematic. *See* Systematic review.
Robust evidence base, in nursing. *See* Systematic review/

S

Synthesis, in systematic review of health care evidence, 468–470
Systematic reviews, of health care evidence, **461–473**
   definition, 461
   difference from other reviews, 461–462
   in mental health, **525–531**
   in pediatrics, **493–506**
   in perioperative care, **485–492**
   in public health, **533–544**
   in rehabilitation, **507–524**
   steps in, 464–472
      framing the question, 464–465
      integrating the findings, 470–472
      looking at quality of evidence, 468
      searching for the evidence, 465–468
      synthesizing the evidence, 468–470
   types of, 463
   uses of, 462–463
   where to find reviews, 463–464
 role in evidence-based health care, **453–460**
   Campbell Collaboration, 457
   emergence in the US and internationally, 454–457
   steps in, 457–459
 trends in publication of nursing-relevant, 477–483
   bibliographic trends in nursing, 479–482

Cumulative Index to Nursing and Allied Health Literature, 479–481
finding reviews, 477–478
gaps in, 483
Joanna Briggs Institute Library, 481–482
overview of, 447–479

T

Translation science, translating evidence into policy and practice, **555–566**
    case study, 558–561
        evidence synthesis, 561–562
        evidence transfer, 562–563
        evidence utilization, 563–564
    translational health cycle, 556–558